TASTY FREEDOM

How We Mastered Fear, Illness and Foreign Travel

with Severe Food Allergies

By Jaquy Yngvason and Josh Greenfield

Tasty Freedom
by Jaquy Yngvason and Josh A Greenfield

Published by Tasty Freedom Inc.
International Standard Book Number:

Printed in the United States of America

Cover Designed by
Nikki Kurt

Edited by
Lisa Willis

This book is dedicated to my father, may he rest in peace. Dad, you always knew that my greatest struggles would be transformed into my greatest strengths so that I could help others who need guidance in their lives to overcame any obstacles they face. Thank you for always believing in me.

~ Jaquy

Table of Contents

Introduction

As much as I would like to say that traveling with food allergies is easy, I'm not going to sit here and lie to you. Truth be told, living with food allergies can be enough of a challenge on its own, but hitting the road, getting out of your comfort zone, flying far away from your kitchen and that local market you love with the little gluten free section, well, let's just say it's enough of a challenge to make me want to write this book. Before we dive right into my life changing trip to Vietnam with my now husband, I figured it would be best to let you know a little bit about me and why I had a burning desire to share this particularly story with you.

While life would have been much easier as a child had I known about the numerous food allergies that I had, I can't say I regret my childhood. Was it crazy? Sure. Did I travel the world like a Gypsy, working from the age of 3 with my parents' business, going from place to place, with virtually no stability? Yep. But it truly made me who I am today and that I would never want to change.

As life would have it, my parents were both immigrants and while they were foreigners trying to make it in America, they had the added challenge of being foreign to one another. And so, you can probably imagine that when my mother, a tiny beautiful and fiery woman from Ecuador, met my father, a robust and powerfully present Icelandic man who loved to share his stories and research about Aliens, Fairies, and Government conspiracies, that as much as they loved one another, their marriage didn't create the most stable of households.

I have no doubt in my mind that they loved me and my older brother and sister dearly but they were hellbent on building up their business and having us work for them, even if that meant pulling us out of school for months at a time to research merchandise and travel around the world with hardly a minute's notice.

As wild as that may sound, my story is only just starting to shape up. As a child I was almost always sick, in and out of hospitals, being flown around the world to meet with doctors, Shamans, holistic health coaches, you name it, I did it. I used to get terrible headaches and no one ever knew what was wrong with me. Some said it was brain tumors, others claimed that I had demons trying to possess me. My parents were willing to try anything, no matter the cost, to help me get well. Unfortunately for the better part of my childhood, no matter how much money they spent (and it was a lot), nothing worked.

Years later, to my amazement, we finally found a doctor who suggested that I was gluten intolerant. And over the years, as it became more well known, I was diagnosed with having Celiac Disease as well as being allergic to eggs and being lactose intolerant.

At the time, Celiac Disease, an autoimmune disease that causes severe damage to the intestine whenever someone eats gluten (wheat, rye, barley), was still unknown to most people, heck the word gluten would make waiters run for the hills. When I was diagnosed there was no gluten free section at the market, and often times if I told someone I was allergic to bread they would usually just laugh. But as much as it sucked, part of me couldn't help but laugh too. After all I used to eat whole loafs of bread while drinking a gallon of milk after a 12 egg omelet for breakfast. My husband likes to joke that my body had had enough of my favorite foods and decided it was time to move on, but I know it's not that simple.

What was simple however was giving up the things that I loved, not at first, but after I realized how much better I felt. Cutting out gluten was a life changer, the headaches and crippling pain went away, the stomach aches and diarrhea disappeared and my body started to function properly. But I won't bore you with that, chances are if you are reading this book you already know what happens when you cut out wheat from your diet.

Being diagnosed with only the beginning. What followed was a series of amazing journeys from moving to Iceland for a year, to going to French Culinary School and having to keep an EpiPen around anytime I ate something I shouldn't (which I wouldn't suggest to anyone), to becoming a food stylist and culinary producer at the Food Network and working alongside some of the biggest chefs in the world. I have since left to become a Holistic Empowerment and Health Coach but you can learn more about that in the about section at the end of this book.

Which brings me to our story, the one you came here for, which takes place about two years ago, when my now husband and partner in magical life crime, Josh, and I decided to take nearly a month-long trip to Vietnam. I had always dreamed of going to South East Asia but after a horrible experience in China many years prior, where I couldn't find any food, got very sick and ended up eating mochi rice cakes the entire time, I was afraid of going anywhere near Asia.

Josh and I have taken lots of little trips in the four years that we have known one another; we've been to New Orleans,

Philadelphia, Vermont, Los Angeles, and Montreal, just to name a few. We have had some incredible experiences traveling together, and have done a pretty good job eating well on each and every adventure, even filming and creating content around eating safely on the road. But most of our trips have been rather short, just a week here or a couple of days there and most of the places that we went we knew it wouldn't be hard to find allergy friendly meals.

Traveling together for upwards of a month, in a place where neither of us spoke the language and we knew little about, was something we had yet to explore, but life was speaking to us and Vietnam was calling. I always felt that the true test of a good relationship came when you travel for an extended period of time with one another, especially in a place that is completely unknown to both of you. I should mention here that Josh has no allergies and can, and does, eat pretty much everything that he sees.

That being said, we love sharing meals together and when we do we tend to eat similar foods, but I knew in Vietnam he would want to eat everything his eyes saw. I also knew that it would be extremely trying for me to not slip up, though I had not in many years, and try something at the risk of it not being safe to eat. I knew it wasn't worth it and I wouldn't put myself at risk, but Vietnamese food is known for being some of the best in the world and I hoped I would be pleasantly surprised with the options.

Traveling with food allergies can be an uphill battle at times, but as a couple we have learned how to handle unpleasant dining situations such as; being kicked out of a restaurant because the chef was offended that we would ask to modify his recipes, to being treated poorly by a waiter who thought my allergies were made up, to knowing what to pack incase we couldn't find safe food. We've even gone through various situations where family members didn't take my allergies very seriously and accidentally served me something I am severely allergic too.

Yes, over the years I have had everything imaginable that could go wrong with food, go wrong. But I never let that stop me, no matter how much of a challenge it was at times. I want to share my story as a homage to all of you out there who are afraid to travel due to dietary restrictions, to those who don't think it's possible to visit exotic places and share truly special meals with friends. To anyone that can relate, Tasty Freedom is for you!

Let this book be a guide to show you the ways of allergy free travel, but not boring get by travel, I'm talking bad ass, have the best time of your life, while eating mouthtastic meals with the people you love travel.

Chapter 1:

Chefs Hate Food Allergies

Late one night two years ago, I sat with a friend who I hadn't seen in years in a dark bar riddled by the loud sounds of locals chatting away and bartenders shaking up fancy cocktails. My friend Hector, a trained chef, has made quite a name for himself after he started a very successful pop up restaurant in Brooklyn. As we sipped on our bourbon, chatting about food and what chefs he thought were the top innovators in their class, I started to see and feel a disconnect between my old friend and I.

An old life, one where I knew all the best bars, partied with the top chefs, stuffed my face with anything I could find, and stayed out until the wee hours of the night, were over. Once I started taking my life seriously I had to take a hard look at the people I was surrounding myself with. Hector was a great way, but we were a world apart and meeting up with him reminded me of just how much life had changed.

As he chatted on I did my best to keep up in the conversation but realized that I had little to offer on the topic. Truth be told I had not been to many restaurants in the past year, I didn't know the latest up and coming news about who was opening the next buzz worthy spot, no, my head was somewhere else.

"Have you eaten there yet?! It's supposed to be amazing!" said Hector as he spoke, wide eyed, about some new hip eating club that had recently been getting some exciting noise in the underground food scene.

"No, I haven't, I haven't really eaten anywhere outside my house recently."

"What? Really? But you love going out to restaurants. I remember not that long ago when you could drink and eat anyone under the table, all after putting in a good 12 hours at the Food Network."

"Ha, well, yeah, those days were certainly something but honestly I don't eat out much anymore. Not because I don't enjoy checking out the latest hot spot, but because I truly enjoying cooking my own food much more and besides–I have so many food allergies"

"I can't argue against a good home cooked meal but still, there's so much inspiration out there. Do you ever feel like you're missing out?"

"Of course, I mean, well sometimes I do. But the more I explore food the more that I find out about all the other amazing things going on in the culinary world, like the Food Allergy Expo," I said excited to share my new life with him.

"Food Allergy Expo? Dude, no offense but that sounds awful. A bunch of people getting together to eat shitty allergy free food? God, and I'll bet you can't travel anywhere because it's too dangerous! And even if you did go, who would want to go with you? Where would you eat? I mean, it already sucks in our friendship!" he said with a half serious laugh.

Hector had an honest, no filter, kind of way about him that I always appreciated, I wasn't much different after all.

"Really, dude?" I said, looking at my supposedly open minded chef friend in shock and disbelief, "you know, you are a good friend, but seriously sometimes you really challenge me to re-evaluate our friendship. If I split open your head, I bet ya I would only find a rock inside," I said, as we both started to laugh. My past work in restaurants gave me a harsh way with words and being with Hector brought back out that quality in me.

"Aw, come on, you love me! Besides, I'm one of your only friends who will go out to eat with you even though it's not as fun now that you're a vegan on top of not being able to eat gluten," he said throwing his hands up to try and lighten the mood

"Don't get me wrong, you know I used to love me some meat," I said taking another sip of my drink.

"Hell yeah, you used to put down a whole 20-ounce steak yourself, maybe you just had more space without all of that bread in your stomach," he said with wide eyes as though he was remembering a time when I put him, and the other boys at the dinner table to shame.

"Haha, yeah but I don't miss meat anymore. Although who knows, I can't say I won't be eating some when Josh and I head to Vietnam next month."

"Woah, whoa, head to where? Did you just say Vietnam? The land of meat, eggs and thanks to the French, a place that has developed a strong love for wheat?"

"Uh, yeah, did you not hear me properly or something?"

"Let me get this straight, you and your boyfriend are traveling to Vietnam together? That sounds like a miserable idea! What are you going to eat there? You don't speak the language, you don't eat meat, fish sauce is in everything, they could poison you, you could die!"

"Wow, thanks for the positive encouragement dude, let me tell you…" I said with a nervous laugh. Maybe he was right, maybe I was making a bad choice. No, screw that! I wasn't going to let his fear- or anyone else's, get in my way.

"I'm just saying…"

"I know, you and everyone else. I can feel the fear, but that must mean that you care, right?"

"It's just that I know what happened when you went to China last time; getting glutenized or whatever the hell they call it, being extremely sick, having to live off mochi for weeks, it sounded miserable. Do you really want to go back into a similar situation?"

"It's something that I'm passionate about, and it's on my bucket list to go to Vietnam. I want to explore and expand my food knowledge, you of all people know how important it is to get out there and learn from other cultures. I'm sick of living in fear, sure I'll need to plan a little bit more than the average person but it's well worth the trip."

"Whatever. I mean, it's your life."

Which brings me to my first little nugget of wisdom I took away from this trip even before I went on it. True, I have lots of food restrictions, but I'm as addicted to exploring new food cultures as any other chef or foodie out there, so why should I feel held back? Living in fear won't get you very far. It's your life, so you need to treat it with a precious kindness and be smart, but with a little creativity and some extra prep work, you can find safe food literally anywhere. I just didn't know it yet, but I was prepared to find out.

"You are so stubborn," said Hector. "I guess I can't stop you, especially if your boyfriend is on board. But man,"

"Listen. I get it, you aren't the first person to call me crazy. But this is bigger than you and me. There are so many people out there who are too afraid to travel the world with food allergies, just like I was. It's high time I show them the ins and outs of how to do it, not in fear, not feeling like a burden, but how to have the best damn time and eat like a queen."

"Hey Pal," said Hector. "I admire your craziness and attitude. I wish you the best of luck, I really do, but if you happen to accidentally eat some wheat and croak, can I have your chef's knives? I always did love that seven inch... Will you, like, have your man leave those for me, or put them in your will?"

We both started to laugh uncontrollably.

"You're sick, you know that? Heck no! They are way too nice for you; with your half assed skills you'll only screw up the edge!"

I think to a lot of chefs that can eat anything, the idea of being restricted by certain foods is almost somehow offensive on such a deep level. The very idea of not being able to cook with butter is somehow damaging to their soul. But I don't blame them, I used to be in a similar boat. Of course, my body paid the price, but as I began to see how stubborn I had been, refusing to listen to what my entire being was trying to tell me- I started to wise up and it made all the difference.

Prior to our trip to Vietnam I did as much research as I could on traveling with food allergies but I came up short. Instead of finding inspiring information and fun tips, I mostly came up with negativity and fear based advice about traveling to South East Asia with food allergies.

I spent hours and hours, googling things like *"Traveling to Vietnam with Food Allergies,"* and *"Being Gluten Free in Vietnam,"* but there was little to be found. Sure, I came across a few blogs here and there about places to eat out that offered options the gluten free traveler, I also found a few things to avoid and things to be careful about, but it wasn't very inspiring, nor did it give me the tools I needed to feel good about making the trip.

But lucky for me I love a good challenge, I find it pushes me creatively and always leads to a wealth of growth. So, I did as much research as I could, found and printed out translation cards for my allergies, packed a little mini traveling "kitchen" in my backpack that had all the essentials and then took some time to pack any protein powder and other basic foods to have in the unlikely event that I really couldn't't find any food.

#Tip: Having little snacks and things to safely munch on is a great way to avoid risking eating the wrong thing when you are really hungry. Sometimes we make the worst decisions when our belly starts to rumble and our hunger takes over. Avoid that by packing little protein bars, nuts, small snacks and dried fruit just in case you can't find anything.

I spent a lot of time in my preparation, almost to the point of mad woman, researching the local food in Vietnam. It was clear that they had a lot of access to great produce and I hoped that finding ways to cook in our hotel room would be easy enough. We had plans to try and find an AirBnB wherever we want but at the time it wasn't yet that popular in Vietnam. Vietnamese cooking is simple in some ways, yet incredibly complex in others. They have a special appreciation for the balance of flavors, often taking a Ying and Yang approach to foods. The food in Vietnam is extremely fresh and fragrant but unfortunately for me, even though they have a lot of gluten free options and rarely use any dairy, finding something without fish sauce or meat was going to be my biggest challenge.

As I sat at my computer, reading through every website that had any mention of gluten free foods in Vietnam an Idea hit me. *I was going to be with Josh, the human garbage disposal.* I would not be alone on this journey; the love of my life would be with me and he too is a chef and arguable more obsessed with food than I am.

Josh, unlike me, can eat everything and also happens to be very good at tasting something and knowing how to make it. I asked him if he would be okay with trying any food that looked good and then helping me recreate allergy free versions once we got back to our room. He, who was always up for a challenge, was thrilled by the idea and we started looking up the local delicacies in every city that we would be visiting.

I knew it was going to be a challenge regardless since Vietnam is known for having some of the best food in the world, most of which I would be unable to eat; really cheap and incredibly well-crafted street food, mouthwatering Pho for $1, the freshest rice noodles with all sorts of curries and stews, whole fried fish, snails, grilled meats- Sounds delicious but I wasn't prepared to go there again, I wasn't going to risk my heath trying something that I was unsure about.

Regardless, I was definitely taking a risk, but it felt right. I knew I couldn't spend my life boxed in in my apartment in Brooklyn, living in fear of the allergy food boogieman. And besides, this time I wasn't alone, I had a supportive partner who was patient with me and always made me feel included when we were eating. Josh and I would conquer this together; I would not be alone.

As the trip neared our anticipation and excitement was growing. We began researching cities that we wanted to visit, we created a loose plan but only really had the first few days mapped out. We were taking in as much information as we could, gathering the gear we needed, as we had planned to film as much of the trip as we could, and then suddenly, out of nowhere, it hit me- I started to feel extremely terrible, sicker than I had been in years. My entire body began to ache and I had absolutely no energy. I hadn't eaten anything wrong and I had no idea what was going on with my body. The trip was rapidly approaching and for the entire week leading up to our departure I was not getting better at all... something was terribly wrong.

Chapter 2:

How to Ruin Your Trip Before It Starts

After days of scrambling to figure out what was wrong with me, my worries began to multiply. I feared that we had to cancel our trip, a trip that would take us into Vietnam for three weeks, and end in San Diego where I was slated to lecture about traveling with food allergies to hundreds of attendees at the Gluten Free Expo. I had planned to speak about my trip to Vietnam, my preparation, how I managed to have a great experience without ever risking my health, and yet here I was, feeling awful, without a clue as to why. As each passing day crept by without any signs of what was going on, I had to ponder the very real possibility of canning the whole trip.

A few days before the trip Josh was doing some research online about what could possibly be going on, looking, searching for anything. As we scanned back to the days before to think of anything that might be causing my body to shut down completely we finally found a lead. What we discovered was that the recent removal of my IUD birth control that I had had in for years was likely to be the root of the problem. As it turns out, and I can't for the life of me understand why I was never informed of this before, when you have something inside of your body that regulates your hormones taken out, well, all hell tends to break lose.

We found case after case of woman who had the Miranda IUD in for years and when they got it removed they suffered from crazy amounts of weight gain, mood swings, an intense decrease of energy, extreme physical discomfort and pain – everything that I started to experience in the recent days had happened to countless woman before me.

Upon finding this out my panic only shot up, this wasn't some sort of random sickness or health plague that would last a few days, no. Per what I read, it was a good possibility that it could take months for my hormones to balance out and my mood to get back in order.

Not knowing what else to do I called up a woman I had interviewed months before, Dr. Antoine, the owner and head doctor at a prominent Holistic Healthcare Center. I told her what was happening and she enlightened me with a wealth of knowledge about what I had to do to balance my hormones out and get my body back where it needed to be. She said that it wouldn't be easy in general, and attempting to do so while traveling to Vietnam would only make my task much more challenging, but with the right supplements and information I should be able to pull myself together and have a great trip.

I ordered about $200 worth of vitamins and a special protein blend right away. Dr. Antoine was concerned in general that with me being a vegan, I was lacking in certain key protein and felt that I needed to bring a substantial amount of protein and vitamins along with me even if it did fill nearly half of my suitcase. She even wrote me a letter in the unlikely event that I was stopped at customs with huge bags of unidentified white powers and pills. The note was a nice touch but I couldn't help but wonder what they might think had I been stopped for a bag search.

Since we would be backpacking around Vietnam we wanted to keep our traveling as light as possible so we went to REI to search out the perfect bag. After finding something that felt sturdy and had easy access to the main compartment we decided to get a fold up non-stick pan just so we know we had something safe to cook in, even if we had to cook at someone's house.

Aside from all my vitamins and supplements I tried to keep my clothing and other accessories to a minimum.

All in all, my packing list included:
- 5 light t-shirts
- 1 Long Sleeve Shirt
- 3 Tank Tops
- 2 pairs of shorts
- 1 pair of long pants
- 1 cute dress for going out
- 1 pair of light hiking boots
- 1 pair of sandals
- 1 pair of sneakers for running
- 1 sports bra
- small jewelry
- 1 bottle of sunscreen
- 1 set of workout clothing
- 2 regular bras
- lots of underwear
- 5 pairs of socks
- a hat for protection from the sun
- sunglasses

- a belt
- 1 towel
- 1 non-stick cooking pan
- Cooking utensils including; a small strainer, a peeler, chop sticks, a rubber spatula, a small knife
- 1 lighter
- Various sized Ziploc bags, parchment paper and aluminum foil.
- A hefty amount of protein bars, Chia, Protein Powder, vitamins, Flax Seeds, dried fruit and nuts.
- Food allergy translation cards printed out on laminated paper.
- 2 things of Tupperware (that I could reuse) packed with food for the plane.

The packing was really important; this wasn't some throw a bunch of stuff in my suitcase and hope for the best type deal. No, I had to carefully think this whole thing through, consider everything that I would need, what the basics were for cooking, I wanted to keep things light but I wanted to be fully prepared.

For as much as I take advantage of my spacious loft and large kitchen space in Brooklyn, when I broke down everything that I would need, the real essentials, to making a good meal, it wasn't all that much. While it seemed a bit daunting at first, as I started to pack, though I wasn't feeling great, I had an air of excitement brewing inside of me just knowing that I was preparing myself for an incredible trip, and that I would be eating amazing foods, even if I had to make most of them myself.

At this point I should note that I wasn't feeling any better, my entire body felt congested, I was getting dizzy and running out of energy quickly, I felt fat and bloated, and I would burst out into tears at the most random of times. Not the most fun when getting ready to leave home for three weeks on what was supposed to be an awesome adventure of traveling, eating and filming the entire experience.

But having discovered the reasons behind my physical ailments gave this trip a new sense of purpose. My redemption from my last visit to Asia was around the corner only this time I had an added challenge. My partner tried to put a positive spin on it like he always does (bless his soul) and say that if I could successfully make this trip, not only with a long list of food allergies, but with the recent health issues from the IUD removal, then it would only be ever more inspiring for someone with food restrictions who happened to not have their IUD removed before heading to South East Asia. At the time, I nearly told him to blow it out his ass, but little did I know how right he would be. With our suitcases packed to the brim, and my head held relatively high (I still had trouble standing up from the spins), we were off to Vietnam.

Chapter 3:

Flying High

At the airport, we checked in, grabbed our tickets and slowly walked toward the dreadful security line. While a lot of my food was stored in my checked bag I made sure to bring plenty of food for the 24 hours of traveling we were headed into, knowing that I could not trust the airport and airplane food. On top of all the food that I brought I made sure to have plenty of vitamins and protein powder in the worst-case scenario that they lost my bag, I didn't want to be food stranded.

As I walked by the caution signs with pictures of what was legal and illegal to bring on a plane my mind began to race. *I have bags full of unmarked pills, hmm… I guess that doesn't look suspicious, does it? What happens if they need to see into my bag, what will I say? I have the doctors note (which is great to have so foods, pills, etc. are not confiscated by TSA), but would they believe me? Oh no this could get bad, no Jaquy shut up, stop being afraid. Everything you are taking is perfectly legal and necessary for your health, if the security people have a problem you can tell them to blow it out their ass. Well, maybe say that, but in a nicer way. Remember, you've got the doctors note, all should be fine. It's perfectly legit!*

Doctor's notes are great, but in the grand scheme of traveling and travel laws in other countries, you never really know what could happen either way so it's best to be prepared and do your research. There is always that odd sensation of the unknown when you travel abroad, it can be a little scary at times but it's also really quite invigorating, there is a certain trust you start to develop the more you get out and see the world.

In the unlikely event that they did want to see into my bag I had everything labeled and would be more than happy to make them a protein shake to prove my innocence, after all, some of the people at the security checkpoint sure looked like they could use some love in their bellies.

One valuable tip that I learned about traveling on airplanes is that they can never take away any food item from me that is not a liquid. It's a different story once you get in to another country and have to go through customs, then you have to be sure to research each country and see what is and what isn't allowed, though typically they only care about things like fresh fruits, vegetables, seeds, meat, and such, but typically you can bring any solid food on the plane with you.

Sauce however, and I love me some sauce, is a bit of a crap shoot, they may spot it and take it away from you, it's sort of a liquid, sort of food, depending on the thickness of it, but I usually just dress my food before just to be extra safe.

Whenever I get up to airport security I just remind myself that everything is perfectly normal. Sure, maybe in this case traveling with a bag of protein powder, vitamins and a foldable cooking pan is a new sort of normal but I wasn't doing anything wrong so I had nothing to fear. I was just a gal headed off to a country I had always dreamed of visiting.

The truth is sometimes in the past I have been hassled by security but honestly no food has ever been taken away from me, sure sometimes I need to be a little extra confident, not be a pushover, explain to people that I have an autoimmune disease and need that food or I'll be in big trouble. Typically, most people just feel bad for me when I tell them why I bring it with me, maybe they have a friend or family member in the same boat, or maybe they just can't imagine living a life without bread.

Being totally transparent with people at the airport, and anywhere for that matter, is good because honesty does go a long way. You can be a bitch about it, get upset that someone doesn't understand the truth about your health problems, but what good does that do? Why not play on their heart strings a little bit, be open, get them to sympathize with your situation, crack a joke about how *you could* eat the food on the plane but that you don't think the rest of the people on the plane would be happy with you stinking up their bathroom the whole way to Asia. Whatever it might be, don't be afraid to say it like it is, even if you do have to put someone in their place – it's your health and you need to be your biggest advocate.

While writing this book, and documenting the trip on paper was important we also decided to film as much as we could. I had high hopes from the start to capture the full experience of traveling in Vietnam, cooking with locals, teaching fun ways to shop at the market and all, but I was getting worried because my health was not improving all that much and I felt so bloated that I balked at the idea of being on camera at all. Even so, we tried to make the best of it, even if it meant the food would be the real on camera star.

The moment the plane took off we got right to it, from the window seat Josh was being super cute taking short videos of everything that was happening while I was busy getting all my food goodies out as I prepped for dinner. Ahead of time we contacted the airline about my food allergies and requested a gluten free and vegan meal but I was prepared with my home cooked food as I've found that most airlines are not trustworthy in this department.

Sometimes airlines will be able to accommodate, and other times they will not. I can't tell you how many times I have ordered the vegan and gluten free meal only to have a flight attendant roll by and drop a plate of god knows what onto my lap and get upset when I ask if this is a special meal for me.

When dinnertime on the airline rolled around and that magical mystery cart came down our isle the attendant came by to ask if I wanted chicken or beef. I said neither and that they should have an allergy free meal in the back for me. The attendant looked puzzled, she didn't speak English very well and I assumed that the only food I would be eating was my own for yet another airplane meal fail. She quickly hurried to the back of the plane to see if they had anything for me.

The guy sitting to my right murmured something under his breath and made a gesture as though he was annoyed that I was attempting to explain to the flight attendant that I needed a special meal. I glanced over at him as though to say "Did you say something? No, I think not." And then, thinking better of it, realizing that it was going to be a long flight and it was best to try and make conversation I simply said "Hello."

We started talking as he began to pull back the tinfoil on the small package in front of him which revealed some sort of beef and broccoli stir fry with rice and a little sweet treat, while I not so patiently waited for my meal to come out. At this point I was all about ready to give up on any chance that they would have a meal ready for me, but I waited in case they did so that I could save my prepared food for later.

As my neighbor stuffed his face, he spoke about how gluten-free is such a bullshit trend nowadays, that it's such a fad, and how annoying it is when his friends pretend to be gluten free and make dining out complicated.

He told me that he was a private chef and worked on the red carpet often catering for Hollywood's highest profile celebrities. "Why don't they just come up with a diet called the 'Eating Disorder Diet'?" he said.

I looked him straight in the face and without skipping a beat, I smiled and said, "Listen, I get that you have probably seen it all; being in Hollywood, dealing with high profile, VIP type folks, who make all sorts of claims and jump on and off the hottest food trends, but you have to realize that some of those people actually have serious food allergies that can be life threatening. It's a real thing dude, you might want to start smartening up to it."

He looked at me blankly and said, "Yeah, yeah, I think it's all made up; people just say they're allergic to something so that they don't come off as having an eating disorder."

Wow, I couldn't believe my ears. There were allergy haters everywhere, even 39,000 feet in the sky. I nearly started to shake before Josh grabbed my hand tightly and reminded me to breathe as I caught his calm gaze staring at me, he too heard what was going on. I tried my best to relax but inside I started to boil a little bit, thinking that I might overflow soon with this guy's BV's (bad vibes). *What an ignorant person!* I thought, but then again everyone has their opinion and there isn't much I can do but live my life in a way that feels right for me.

A few minutes later the flight attendant came to deliver my gluten-free, vegan dish, labelled and everything. As I unwrapped my meal I noticed the guy sitting next to me looking at the food and shaking his head, enough was enough, I had to say something.

"Listen dude," I said, "I get that to you this isn't a big deal, and yes a lot of people lie and say that they have food allergies and take advantage of others for it, but one day you just might come to find out that someone you love or care about has a serious food allergy and that your life may turn around because of it. What if you met the love of your life and she was allergic to wheat?"

"Well, I, I."

"What if every time that you ate bread you couldn't kiss her without running the risk of making her sick? What then? Do you know you could put her at serious risk, even just the tiniest amount of gluten, the size of a piece of rice, can make me extremely sick for weeks and cause permanent damage to my gut."

"Woah, I had no idea. It just seems like a fad; most people don't even know what gluten is."

"I hear you dude, a lot of people are ignorant to it but it only makes it harder for those of us that seriously suffer. Do you know how many times I've heard of people gluten poisoning their partner secretly just because they didn't believe that they had a food allergy?"

"Really? That is crazy."

"I know, which is why this is no joke dude."

"Wow, thank you for sharing that, I really had no idea, I've got to rethink this whole thing, I'm sorry about that."

"No sweat. Listen, it happens, even with my family. I had to go through this for years.

I'm glad I could calm myself because I nearly blew my lid on this guy. I won't pretend I don't have the temper to do so, being half Latin and all, but what good would that have been? Sure, I could have screamed at him for being a jerk, it would have felt good for a few seconds, stooping down to a level below my own. But in the end, I would only be doing a disservice to myself. Instead I just told him the truth, shared a bit about my experience's and struggles with food allergies, related it back to him in a way that he might be able to empathize with. In the end, I think he heard my message loud and clear. By opening up that space for yourself and being real, you'd be amazed what can come out of it.

I do find it interesting how people perceive different food allergies. For instance, one time we were on a plane getting ready to take off and the flight attendant buzzed in on the intercom to inform everyone that they would not be serving peanuts on the flight and to please avoid eating any peanuts as someone on the plane had a serious peanut allergy. Instead of the peanuts they would be serving pretzels and crackers.

"That's odd isn't it," said Josh.

"What do you mean?" I replied a bit confused.

"Well I get why they are not serving peanuts of course, peanut allergies are extremely serious, but they've just taken away the one snack that you are not allergic too."

And that's just it, peanut allergies are taken seriously as they should be because people can get seriously sick and even die from eating a small number of peanuts. However, what most people don't know is that you can die from eaten gluten if you have Celiac Disease as well. It isn't an instant, call an ambulance, sort of thing, but something that slowly over time can cause you to have any number of terminal illnesses all because your body isn't getting the proper nutrition.

When I finally did open my mystery meal that was supposedly safe for me to eat I had to take a moment to pause and consider what I was doing. Anything not prepared in my own home or a dedicated gluten free kitchen runs the serious risk of cross contamination, so I must be very careful.

While you can never be too safe, one thing that I have learned over the years is to trust my gut, after all it is the thing that will be directly affected if I eat the wrong thing. Josh calls me the "Bullshit detector." Whenever we walk into a restaurant and ask about whether or not they can accommodate my food allergies I can tell within seconds whether I will be eating there.

If I feel safe when I talk to the wait staff or chef, if they take my allergies seriously, ask me questions and talk to me about it, or share with me how they deal with this all the time or that they know someone that has food allergies and are aware of how serious it is, then I feel comfortable and like I am in good hands. But on the other hand, if they don't take it seriously, if they don't know what is in the food or won't take a few minutes to go find out, or worse – act annoyed, well, then we high tail it out of there.

When it came to eating the meal on the plane I was very thorough about asking whether the food was safe or not. I am never afraid to tell someone that if the food in front of me has anything I am allergic to in it, I will get very sick and have to go to the hospital. This usually wises them up real fast.

In the end, I ate the meal, the hostess was very nice and assured me, once I busted my allergy cards out, that it was perfectly safe and good to eat. And good it was indeed, surprisingly good, even Josh said he had wished he had put in for a gluten free and vegan meal, fresh steamed broccoli, carrots and a little rice. Add that to some of the food that I had already prepared and I was already on my way to food paradise. Delicious meal number one, check!

Chapter 4:

<u>Feeling Like a Drug Smuggler at Customs</u>

The moment we got off the plane in Vietnam it was hot, I mean real hot, as if I had walked into a steam room, all my clothes clung to me as though they were hanging on for dear life. At first it was nice to get out of the airplane, stepping away from the circulated air where my mind raced with paranoia about what might be floating around in it, but then I just felt gross as my body began to sweat.

We followed the crowd to the migrations area and had to get our Visa prepared. Before we left we did a lot of research about the best way to get a Visa to get into Vietnam. As it turns out there are two main ways to do so. For one you can either get a visa through the Vietnamese Embassy, fill out some forms, pay a bit over $100, send in your passport, wait to get it back and then be on your way. This way was more expensive but once you got into the country, you simply presented the Visa at customs and you were good to go.

The second way was to obtain a visa is to get a "Visa Upon Arrival," where you fill out a simple form online, pay less money, get a small piece of paper guaranteeing you entry and then when you get into Vietnam you have to pay a little more money and you get your visa right at the airport. It saved us money to do it that way, though it felt a little riskier, in the end it was quite easy and the only difference was about a 30-minute delay waiting at the airport to get the paperwork. It turns out most travelers who frequent Vietnam did the same, so we felt good about our decision.

Josh had also done some research (as I was feeling too out of it leading up to the trip from my IUD fiasco to help) on getting through customs. He had done less world traveling than I had and was a little concerned from the stories that he had read online about the Vietnamese customs officers giving people a hard time. I'm sure it wouldn't't have been as concerning but the last thing either of us wanted was for me to have to forfeit the hundreds of dollars' worth of protein powders and vitamins I had purchased specifically to stay healthy on this trip.

Josh told me that through his research he had learned that some people had issues getting through customs. I could tell he was a little bit concerned, but myself, being accustomed to traveling around the world since I was a child, typically didn't think much about customs. Today however I wasn't feeling well, and it was a full day of travel, so I started to get nervous. He read reviews about how some people had complained that customs officers would want to look through their stuff thoroughly, sometimes taking things out and keeping them for themselves for no good reason, he even read that some of them required bribes to get through.

When we got to the front of the line at customs, we did our best to breath slowly and relax, being sure not to show any nervousness if there was any going on inside. The customs officer looked very serious and hardly said a word to the other travelers as he checked their passports one by one. When we were called up to the customs officer we immediately presented our passports, and I, in typical Jaquy fashion, tried to be friendly and ask him how he was doing. Without even ever looking up at us he simply stamped our passport and we were on our way in seconds.

As we later learned, foreigners never had issues getting through customs, it was actually the locals that the officers would often give a hard time to. For whatever reason, they openly welcomed foreigners coming through but from time to time would cause issues and demand bribes from locals trying to get back into the country.

When we got out onto the street it was late, somewhere around 2 am, the air was hot and dry, but it felt fresh after being inside for the past 24 hours. On top of already not feeling great I was extremely tired and jet lagged and seeing the whirling lights and hearing the chaotic sounds of the airport made me feel like I was in the movie Speed, I needed to get to a cab fast before I lost it.

We got into one of the safe cabs (they are green and white) and showed the cab driver a print out of the name of the hotel we were staying at. The cab driver took one look at the directions to our hotel and just started driving like a mad man, without saying anything at all to us. Josh had this look on his face, and I, feeling the panic in his eyes, took a deep breath and reached for his sweaty hand to hold it tight.

"We are okay," I whispered to him, "It's just the way it is here."

I almost gave in to his slight sense of fear but my heart knew that we were taken care of, that we made it this far, and that all was well. It was just those beginning of the trip jitters and a bit of culture shock, no big deal. I find that whenever I travel to a foreign place there is always going to be a little fear, whether it be my own or the person I am traveling with. While it may be off putting at first, this is perfectly normal. I mean, come on, you are traveling to a distant land where no one speaks your language, you can't expect to just fit right in the second you get there, it takes time to adjust. Besides, that's all part of the fun!

Josh had booked us a little hotel in the heart of Ho Chi Minh by the backpackers' district. We had found great prices on Agoda and figured it was our best but unless we should meet someone who tells us otherwise. It would have been nice to find a place with a kitchen early on but we knew we would be staying at a variety of spots and a hotel was a great first destination, it was in a busy area, it had a person at the desk that we could get information from and it was simple.

When we pulled up to the hotel it was nearly 3 am. The street was lined with people drinking and laughing the night away. We saw bright lights, smelled scents we had never experienced before, it was all quite exciting, even with the jet lag. We saw street performers, and food carts everywhere our eyes could see, I heard the loud thumping of base through the car, and I started to feel a little better, I felt right back in New York City. Maybe we're not going to get chopped up into tiny little pieces and tossed in some soup. [Insert nervous laughter]. Amazing where the brain can go off little sleep in a foreign place right?

The taxi driver abruptly stopped in front of our hotel and gestured for money. We pulled out some American dollars as we had yet to have a chance to convert our currency and began pointing to the different sized bills. We had heard that the drivers would accept the dollar but that they might over charge. Luckily, we knew that the price was somewhere around $5 and he seemed okay with that.

We got out of the taxi and looked out at the door infant of us, it didn't quite look like a hotel but we saw a small dinky sign by the door with the name. When grabbed our things and walked towards the tall glass front door of the hotel lobby that was next to a loud bar. The smells of street meat, spices and herbs was truly pungent and intoxicating, in the most beautiful way. I could already see Josh eyeing the small street carts being pushed around by a few older women who seemed to have not a care in the world.

When we got to the door it looked like the hotel was closed and we started to freak out a little bit. The lights were off, no one was around, and on top of that it looked like some of the guests were literally sleeping on beds in the lobby. What the hell was happening? Was this all a dream? Had I not really been sick, were we indeed back in Brooklyn?

As we knocked, lightly at first as to not disturb whoever was sleeping, no one answered. Were we stuck, at 3am, with all our personal belongings, alone, without a phone, and a wad of cash in our money belt on the streets of Vietnam?

Just then we saw some movement as a medium statured Vietnamese male who worked at the hotel quickly jumped up from underneath the covers of a blanket on the lobby couch. Looking closer we realized that he and his colleague were sleeping in the lobby, one on the couch and another on a pull-out bed. For a moment, I felt kind of bad for waking them up and then quickly realized that this was a hotel and it probably wasn't a big deal.

The door opened and the one guy spoke in a broken English. "Come in, come in, please."

"Thank you, we were getting worried there," I said.

"Please, I need credit card and passport, yes, I need now then I show you to your room," he said calmly but firmly.

He took us to our room which was nothing like the photo on the website claimed it to be, it was small, had no air conditioner or window, and it smelled strange. I looked at Josh and said, "Babe, we can't sleep here. It's smaller than a closet, and the bathroom is down the hall!" Josh asked him if there was anything else.

"I swear, babe, I'm not being a diva," I said. "It's just I *feel super* claustrophobic in here. I just can't do it.

The hotel worker seemed confused and was getting ready to leave, assuming we were about to settle into our room but I looked at him and asked where the room in the picture was with the big window and the bathroom.

When he finally understood, what I was trying to say he took us to another room but told us that it would cost a lot more.

"How much more is it going to be?" I said. "We paid for a different room than the one you are showing us." "Eight," he said. Eight, of course, eight more dollars, I nearly forgot how cheap Vietnam was.

We went up one floor and entered a room that had a huge window, air conditioning, a private bathroom, a large bed and a mini fridge. Jackpot! This was the room we had booked and while I could have fought for no price increase it would only cost us a whopping $24 a night. There was however one small issue.

Turns out we were staying right near the backpacker district in Ho Chi Minh city, a very touristy, but safe, area and as we came to find out, an area that never really sleeps, hence the drunk people out on the streets at 3am. It would be noisy throughout the night, but at least we had a bigger room and window, and besides I brought my ear plugs so I would be able to shut out the world around me.

After we put our stuff down and settled in I immediately went to take a shower. Though it wasn't a shower like the one I am used to, it felt great. It was a little odd seeing as how there was no sink, just a small open bathroom with a toilet and a shower head next to it. And so, you can imagine to my "delight" that the toilet paper was soaking wet after my shower There is however nothing quite like washing off after hours of travel in a hot country. The refreshing rinse made me start to feel like myself again and though I should have been ready to pass out I could tell that Josh wanted to go out and explore, he looked hungry, and I didn't want to be alone without him just yet.

We headed out to the bustling street and everywhere we looked there was something going on; crazy drunk college students stumbling, laughing, eating, tourists wandering the streets searching for their hotel, old women working away at large food carts followed by a line of hungry pedestrians.

It was a sight unlike anything that I had ever seen before. Everywhere I looked it felt like we were on an Anthony Bourdain show, although unlike Bourdain, I would not be the ballsy eat-anything-I-see-on-the-streets kind of gal, but I liked taking in the sights none the less.

Between working at the Food Network, going to culinary school, and being food obsessed, this was the dream. To come to a place bustling with bubbling pots of delicious broths, simmering meats, noodle salads being tossed mid-air, it was a symphony of food being orchestrated by masters of the meal right before our very eyes. As much as I wished I could eat everything in that moment, I couldn't help but feel content simply admiring the craft as though it was an ever-changing collection of art.

I turned around for what felt like a second to see if any convenient stores were open and before I knew it Josh was learning over an old woman's ladle and taking a taste of the unidentified rice porridge before him.

I panicked, "Babe! What are you doing? You have to be careful, you can't just eat from some random person on the street's spoon. He just shrugged and smiled, completely unfazed by my concern, put up his finger to the woman, gesturing that he would like one bowl, and came back with a big grin on his face.

"Sweetie, I love you but you have to be careful," I said.

"Relax," he said. "It's all right, besides, she let me try it right off her spoon! It's really tasty and I can't hold back, there is just so much amazing food here, and I want to try it all!"

Oh man, not only was I dealing with my own health issues, but I began to fear that I might be soon dealing with his if he wasn't more careful about what he ate on the street. I love him to death but sometimes he can be a little too reckless and it scares the crap out of me.

Having traveled the world with my parents from a young age I have learned a lot about the ins and outs of street eating. The cart that Josh just hit looked like stomach issues central! Before I started to rant all about it he must have known it was coming because he just smiled at me and said, "I know what you're going to say, but there's no way that I'm going to get sick. It was just too good, I know what I'm doing, you gotta trust me love."

I just looked at him and chuckled nervously, "I know, I love you, I just don't want you to get sick is all."

I didn't end up eating anything that night as I was still stuffed from the food that I had brought on the plane. Really I just wanted some water and sleep. Besides, I wasn't ready to take a chance eating out until I knew I had a clear rested mind and could make smart choices.

We got back to our room and fell right into bed, clothing and all, sweaty and smelling of street essence. We quickly fell asleep to the thumping bass that shook our whole room with its rumbling vibrations. Therapeutic really, calming in an odd way, if you enjoy that sort of thing. Or maybe I have been living in New York City for too long.

★Street Cart Safety Tips★

I know there is a tendency to want to go on the see food diet. You see it and you eat it. However, when eating on the street, I advise you to consider the following.

1. Is the person handling the food wearing gloves? If so, this is a good sign.

2. Is there more than one person working the cart? It's a good sign if you order from a cart where one person is doing all the cooking and someone else is handling the money exchange.

3. Is there a long line? If you see a busy cart, especially one busy with locals this is usually a good sign that the cart is safe, popular and delicious.

4. How does the food look? If the food looks fresh and clean that is a good sign, same goes for the person working the cart, if they are clean and seem put together that is a good tell.

5. Where is the meat in relation to the other food? Is there meat on the cart? Is it raw? If the meat is raw is it anywhere near the vegetables?

6. Try not to over eat. I know there is a tendency to want to eat everything and eat it fast, but take your time with the food, eat slow, savor it, sit down and eat, get comfortable, don't just shove the food down your throat.

7. What sort of feeling do you get from the cart? This is important, overall how do you feel waiting in line or standing near the cart. At the end of the day you can only pray for the best, and you must know that eating at any street cart poses some potential risk, though typically it is usually just the runs, you want to be careful and trusting your gut is a great way to do so.

For me, eating the wrong thing means being sick for weeks and having several future complications, so regardless of these tips I still have to be extra careful and you do too if you have food allergies. Your safest bet is finding a cart that sells only things that you are not allergic too.

For example, I wouldn't eat from any place that made Banh Mi because of the bread. I would however highly consider eating at a stall that just served steam corn or sweet potato. Most of the people working these carts get up early every morning, shop for fresh ingredients and cook everything either at home or more often right at the cart so you know they are only really working with what you see. Another good note, look around at the ingredients, often times a street vendor only makes and sells one or two things and you can very visibly see everything. It's still important to ask and flash your translation cards, but every little thing helps you in making an educated guess.

I don't eat meat or fish by choice but it won't make me sick so getting a little fish sauce or meat juice in my food isn't the end of the world. It's not something I would do back home but if a delicious dish was calling to me, I might let it slide here or there so as to not pass something up along my journey.

While I had to be extra careful of what I ate, Josh, having no food allergies, still had to be leery of "Traveler's Diarrhea." I am not pretending that this is his only threat— there are other potentially dangerous illnesses that you must be careful of, but often, travelers fall victim to Traveler's Diarrhea and are plagued by not being able to keep any food down for a few days which can lead to malnourishment and dehydration. On top of ruining a few days of your trip.

I did my best to educate Josh, even scare him a little. I'm not saying I'm proud of it but my parents were no different with me. I wanted him to be careful and watch what he ate, but there was only so much that I could share with him. We were both in a foreign country and he had to make his own decisions. Even so that didn't stop me from attempting to guide his sometimes-stubborn-ass from time to time. I love him to death but sometimes his carefree attitude scares the crap out of me.

Chapter 5:

Phogive Me for I Have Skimmed

The next morning I woke up and, forgetting that we were in a hot hotel room in Vietnam, felt like someone had peed all over me. I was sticky, hot and covered in sweat, I could hardly move. What had happened to me in the past 24 hours?

Before I got out of bed, Josh came over smiling and excited like he had a sweet secret to whisper into my ear. He was already dressed, full of energy and as he leaned in to kiss me he said with a great big grin "Holy amazing! We are in Vietnam!"

"Haha. We are?" I said. "I feel like shit, like I don't want to move. Why am I feeling like this?"

Suddenly I burst into tears and Josh gave me huge hug, telling me it was all right, assuring me that I was just jet lagged and that a cold shower would make it all better.

I got up, undressed myself and got in the shower while Josh went out to find us some fresh fruit for breakfast and exchange some currency. As the water bounced off my legs I looked down and noticed that my arms and legs were incredibly swollen, I felt like I was the size of an elephant and I immediately burst into tears, what the hell was wrong with me?

I cried my eyes out for a few minutes and slowly settled into the very present possibility that the entire trip, my trip that was supposed to be the best, one to check off my bucket list, might very well be plagued by my health condition. Sure, I was prepared to eat safely, but my hormones were out of control and I had no idea what to do.

When Josh got back he had a look on his face of raw excitement. He had just been to some fresh fruit stalls and got the most beautiful mango, dragon fruit and bananas that I had ever seen, and they all only cost about $1. We ate fresh fruit with chia pudding that I made from some hot tea. I asked the hotel for a water kettle and they gladly provided one for us. We didn't have any heating sources yet but little things like boiling water can really go a long way.

We made a beautiful rainbow chia salad parfait with the fresh and vibrant fruits that was both invigorating and amazing. I whipped up a little chocolatey mint breakfast drink made by adding chocolate protein powder to mint tea. Our peeler, cutting board and small knife was already going a long way. I was starting to feel better just sitting there enjoying our fresh breakfast. The fruit was literally to die for, the flavors exploded on my tongue, it reminded me of when we would visit my Mom's family in Ecuador.

After a good healthy breakfast, I got changed and we walked outside, Vietnamese currency (the Dong) and allergy free cards in hand, ready to explore. At first I was reminded of that "lovely" feeling of my arms and legs peeing sweat all over me but after thirty minutes or so it didn't seem to bother me anymore. I was stinky, but hey, who cares, it was hot and we were in heaven.

I kept thinking about how I could possibly clog the pores of my armpits so that I wouldn't feel like Pepe Le Pew (natural organic deodorant is not your friend in this climate). My internal bitching kept going on and on but as we walked through the city streets, past a park and towards a few Pho restaurants, the chatter in my brain slowly started to let up.

After walking around and exploring for a bit we wanted to give our allergy free cards a shot, and I just wanted my first bowl of Pho, so we headed to a spot we had read about called Pho 24. In preparation for our trip we did as much research as we could about safe places for me to eat and though there wasn't much, this was one place that they said was safe for anyone with celiac disease.

When we got inside we walked up to the workers there and showed them my allergy card stating that I could not eat anything with gluten; wheat, rye or barley, nor could I eat any meat products, seafood, eggs, or dairy. The waiter studied the cards for a long time before looking back at us with an apologetic and confused face.

He smiled politely and said, "No, no…we no, no."

It seemed that even though wheat wasn't a problem, they did not have any vegetarian options. *Shit, I hope the next place has something.*, I thought. *Why did my body have to stop liking meat?* Oh well, let's sally forth!

We left Pho 24 and headed next door to Pho 2000, another spot that we were told had gluten free Pho, with a little less confidence than we had originally ventured out with. Both places were fast food restaurant chains specializing in Pho and even though I wanted something super authentic I was willing to settle for anything safe to start. After all, chain or not, it was going to be more authentic than any Vietnamese food I had ever had before, I mean we were in the place that invented the dish.

When we showed our allergy cards to the waiter, he looked them over for a few minutes and then shot us a confident glare. He smiled, nodded his head and said, "Yes, yes, yes, sit, yes. Come right this way."

Boo yakasha!! We made it! *Maybe there is hope for me in Vietnam after all*, I thought. I just have to keep my hope up and my confidence strong—of course I wasn't the first person to visit this country with food allergies, there is an awareness here, I could feel it.

My first chance to try real traditional Vietnamese food, I was thrilled and Josh was thrilled too, we could not wait to eat! However, let me make this very clear: I was still not committed to eating the food. I always abide by the rule of three. I had to wait and see if it was safe for me to eat and I was prepared to walk away if I felt any bit of doubt creep in.

★Tips for Eating Out: Rule of Three★

1. When you first arrive at a restaurant ask the manager or wait staff if they can safely accommodate you.

2. Once you are seated talk to manager or waiter to confirm that what you are ordering is completely safe and that they understand you could get very sick if not. Don't be afraid to seem a little bit annoying or come off as high maintenance, you must take your health into your own hands. As a matter of fact, sometimes it's good to be a little crazy (not too much) because then the staff seem to take it seriously.

3. When the food arrives, triple check and ask the waiter and/or manager if your food is safe once again and check to make sure that they brought the right dish to you.

4. This isn't exactly part of the rule of three but whenever I get food delivered to me I always take a minute to set an intention and bless the food, clearing it of any unwanted negative energy that may otherwise enter my body. Taking a moment to make sure that your mind is in the right place when you sit down to eat can surprisingly make all the difference.

As we sat patiently waiting to talk to the waiter who would be serving us, we noticed a huge picture of Bill Clinton on the wall eating at the restaurant. Apparently, it has become somewhat of a tourist attraction ever since the former president had graced his mouth with their hot and steamy bowl of noodles!

We looked over the menu and were pleased to see that it had an English translation side to it. This really helped to identify whether the restaurant served any wheat or something else that I was allergic too.

Since some places serve Banh Mi, something that in America we consider a sandwich on a long baguette stuffed with meat and all sorts of delicious stuff (but in Vietnam it just means bread), this is always going to be your biggest challenge. Because of the French influence, there is a lot more wheat in Vietnam than we expected but even so, Vietnam's major export crop is rice and you can almost guarantee to see mostly rice-based menus wherever you go. Luckily for us Pho 2000 didn't have anything wheat on the menu; it was just pure Pho and traditional soups. Score!

Even though it was a gluten free spot, it's even more reason for someone to be extra careful. When you have celiac disease or any dangerous food allergies you don't want to think to yourself, *Hey, its gluten free, I am all set!* I've known the feeling but there are other factors to consider, like some rice noodles can be made with wheat so you want to be sure to ask about that.

It is always better to ask than to assume. We ran into a few situations where we saw what seemed to be fresh and pure rice noodles but found out that they had a small amount of wheat in them.

Good news though, in Vietnam everyone seems to have a deep love and respect for food and tend to know exactly what is in their products. Most of the meals we came across were super fresh and easy to identify. Processed food doesn't seem to be as big of a thing in Vietnam as it is in the states. But again, be careful.

As a vegan, another thing I had to keep an eye out for was fish sauce and MSG. Though I am not allergic to meat I don't very much want fish sauce in my food, and I don't feel well when I eat MSG, it makes my throat feel itchy and it makes me dizzy.

Being gluten free is one thing but being vegan in Vietnam is a whole other thing. No meat, no fish sauce, (which is in nearly everything), no eggs-that was the challenge. Dairy wasn't much of an issue as they use very little of it, but on top of the no wheat, I was rather limited even in my gluten free options.

When I would be speaking to a waiter I would say, "Vegetarian only" and they would point to fish! It was always comical because to them beef and pork are what they consider meat so I can understand their recommendation of fish as a vegetarian option. Dieting and food allergies were not all that prevalent but the allergy cards were truly a life saver.

★Fish Sauce Tip★

Most fish sauces are gluten free but not all. And while it is unlikely if you are unsure don't be afraid to request the bottle to check for yourself as fish sauce is used in almost everything. Vietnamese cuisine does however lend itself to personalized additions which was nice. Often you will get a simple bowl of something like a flavorful broth and noodles and at the table have the options to add your chilies, fish sauce and fresh herbs.

Once I made sure that I felt safe we scoured the menu and found that they had a delicious sounding vegetarian Pho that I was eager to try. We showed the waiter our allergy-free cards, but he didn't really speak English, so we started the pointing game.

"Does *this* have *that* in it?" I said.

Confidently he said, "No."

He went on to point out, that there was no "bột mì" (wheat flour) in the whole restaurant. This made me feel super comfortable and safe and I was oh-so-ready to order.

We ordered the vegetarian pho with no fish sauce, and some fresh mango. After we put in our order Josh and I looked at each other with pure elation! It was a nice feeling to have had our first win together, success!

Sitting in triumph and excitement for the delicious meal that would soon be coming, we patiently, or rather impatiently waited as we stared at the bustle of cars and motorbikes zipping by below the restaurant.

As we peered down at the chaos that is any typical Vietnamese street in the city we noticed that there seemed to be no real laws governing the thousands of motorbikes mindlessly racing around the streets. No cars ever seemed to stop for anyone and motorbikes flew by in every direction. Pedestrians confidently walked right through oncoming traffic as the motorbikes swiftly weaved their way around them, it was a magical dance of chaotic beauty.

Before the soup came out the waiter brought us our order of fresh mango and we immediately noticed a problem. The mango was served with crushed ice. To the average person that might not seem like anything but it can be extremely dangerous to drink water as a foreigner when visiting a third world country.

From our research, crushed ice is a problem in Vietnam. With the water filtration system, it was very hard to know whether ice was safe, as most of it was just frozen from tap water. While the locals have the right parasites and bacteria to handle the water that they have grown up drinking, for anyone outside of the country it can make you very sick, often leading to severe diarrhea. I know, I know, gross but true!

While some ice is completely safe, and though it is really tempting to suck back a fresh glass of ice water on an extremely hot day, you should be careful what you drink. It's best to air on the safe side and stick with bottled water.

Ice Tip

Look for ice that is cylinder in shape and has a hole punched through it. These shapes are considered safe because they are made in factories. The shape of ice gives a clear visual if you should or shouldn't be drinking the water that is served to you. If you don't see the shape of the ice then it's probably not worth drinking it. "Khong Da" (pronounced Khom Da) means no ice in Vietnamese.

When we tried to return the fruit, and asked for mango without ice we noticed that there were some translation issues. We quickly realized that we had to learn the translation for no ice fearing that if we did not it would become a problem.

They brought us back some fresh cut up mango with no ice, though we could tell it was probably the same mango, and as we sat in the air-conditioned room with Bill Clinton looking at us, we thought about what a big commitment no ice would be in a hot country during one of it's hottest times of the year.

As we waited, chomping on our mango, we kept looking at the various wait staff bringing out big bowls of soup, hoping that ours would be next. We struck up a conversation with an older gentleman who was visiting his son who had recently moved to Ho Chi Minh, which by the way we found out should be called "Saigon" as the locals prefer to call it.

When the soup finally came out it looked incredible. I was a little bit skeptical because in the states whenever I order Vegetarian Pho they tend to just serve a vegetarian broth with rice noodles and a very small and insignificant amount of vegetables. But no, this was totally different.

The soup was filled with huge pieces of cooked tofu, and a plethora of vegetables galore—it was delectable. But before we ate, and probably at the annoyance of the waiter, we asked one more time if it was allergen free just to be absolutely sure that there was nothing unsafe for me in it.

I even pointed to the "If I have wheat it will make me sick," part of the card. He once again seemed very sure and gestured as though to promise us to relax and that it was all good. Even so, we (as we always do), blessed the food, adding that extra layer of safety to our meal and then quickly dug in to what was our first delicious Pho experience in Vietnam. And boy, was it delicious! Probably the best bowl of Pho I have ever had. This place might be a chain but it was nothing like the chain restaurants back home. It was warm, flavorful, clean, and fresh and my taste buds were exploding with rich flavor. Oh, what a win that was. Life was good, I was already starting to feel like myself again.

Chapter 6:

Local Tourists

After our delicious Pho experience we headed across the street, being as careful as we could not to get struck by one of the many motorbikes that were zipping down the street, to Ben Thanh Market.

Thank god, we were coming from New York, an arguably equally crazy city, otherwise the motorbikes everywhere would have probably freaked us out a bit more. As we waited for a clearing in the traffic which felt like forever, we realized that we just had to go for it. We had to just march forth through oncoming traffic, and hope and pray for the best. Scary as hell at first, but slowly, as we finally worked up the courage to cross the street we realize that it was quite safe.

You just have to be confident and walk straight. Do not hesitate because the motorbikes are used to people crossing the street and will always go around to avoid you, so keep straight on your path, head held high, breath and have some fun- it was such a rush of adrenalin at first.

Ben Thanh Market is famous for its night scene, especially with tourists, it is an incredible night market to visit for your fill of cheap souvenir shopping and food. During the morning and early afternoon hours it's where the locals shop for ingredients and eat, which is precisely our favorite time to go, it's less crowded and we get to feel what it's like for the locals.

We were told to be careful about prices as they are often jacked up for tourists. During the day, Ben Thanh Market houses a ton of little souvenir stalls as well as incredible food and fresh produce, meat and fish.

Walking around the market left us amazed at first, the sheer amount of stuff they had was mind blowing, but our amazement quickly turned into humor as the haggling began. There were thousands of vendors inside, all selling similar stuff: clothing, souvenirs, bowls, cups, plates, bags, wallets, anything that a large market would sell, they had. The thing is they weren't just selling, they were pushing things on us hard. Anytime you made eye contact with someone it was very much a "you buy from me" and "how much you want to pay?" type of interaction. We found ourselves bargaining for stuff that we didn't even want just to see how low we could get them to go before walking away, sometimes accidentally buying something. For us this is always the most exciting and most dangerous time to shop, and they knew that.

When we found the actual food market it was like an indoor farmers' market full of produce stands: fresh meat, vegetables, seafood and fruit. On top of that there were a ton of vendors all selling a variety of Vietnamese cuisine: spring rolls galore, fried this, stuffed and steamed that. It was all a bit overwhelming, I could see Josh, wide eyed, was already ready to eat everything.

The currency at the time was about one U.S dollar to 21,000 Dong, making us feel like absolutely ballers holding millions of Dong in our pockets. The dollar, as we started to see early on, really went a long way. Your average incredible street food meal would only cost you about $1 but as cheap as everything was it was almost a little too cheap, if you know what I mean. Getting this idea that everything was so cheap and that you could buy whatever you wanted started to add up surprisingly quickly. A dollar here and a dollar there could quickly turn into $50 before you even blinked if you weren't careful.

We walked around looking at all the food stalls, I was stuffed from the soup but I knew that Josh wanted to try something and I had no problem exploring with him. We began searching around for what seemed delicious in such a vast market and quickly came across a stall that was packed with locals, far busier than any other spot in the whole place. This, from what we had read, was usually a good sign. Find the places that are busy where lots of locals are eating. You can be sure that the food is damn good, and usually safe too.

It looked as though everyone was eating the same thing but we could not for the life of us, make out what it was. It looked delicious and before I could say anything I saw Josh put his finger up for one. The sign said Banh Beo, it seemed to be really all that they served and as we sat waiting for his meal I noticed fresh coconut water being served and ordered us two. The coconut came out first, green on the outside, delicious and refreshing water on the inside. I have had many fresh coconuts in my life, but boy did we take a liking to fresh coconut water on our trip. They cut it open on the spot, stuck a straw in it and plopped it in front of us. It was cold, refreshing and as we sucked down on our straw we felt the most healing, replenishing, hydrating, soothing, fresh, and incredible liquid course down our throat.

When Josh's food came out it looked really special. This was our first attempt to really dissect the local food. Everyone around us seemed friendly with smiles on their faces as they sat happily eating the dish before them. They would point and make gestures about the food, seeming to be trying to tell me that the food was good and that I should eat it too. They were perceiving our want to dissect the food as a reluctance to eat it.

Josh and I laughed and made some expressive jokes to keep the mood light, to let the locals know that we were not afraid and felt comfortable and relaxed as though we had been in Vietnam for quite some time and they laughed right back at us.

One of our favorite things to do when dining out, especially at a place where I cannot eat, is to have Josh order something that looks good and then we will look at the food, pick it up, move it around, and he will try each thing slowly: the sauce, the garnish, the meat, the dish, noting the textures, the flavors, the balance, the technique. As he eats we will try and figure out what makes it special and what he likes about it. How can we find a way to make this dish safe for me? That was a big part of the mission of the trip: Josh would go out, try something on the street or in a restaurant that I could not eat, and then we would go to the market to do our best to recreate a modified and safe version for me or find a way to make it back home.

Josh ate through his Banh Beo, a delicious looking dish that consisted of steamed rice cakes all filled with different things such as prawns and fish, topped with a fish cake, some crispy garnish, scallions, chili and fish sauce. He said it was awesome but super spicy. He wasn't all that good with super spicy, but it was extremely fresh and delicious, unlike anything that he had ever had in his entire life.

After Josh finished his meal we headed on our way to buy some produce, but before we did I needed to go to the bathroom. (Let's just say I have the world's smallest bladder and seeing as how I had just drank an entire coconut...)

When I entered the bathroom, I noticed something quite odd, yet awesome. A woman, after using the bathroom, was using a hose to wash herself off. It was a hot day and I decided to do the same. I washed my feet, my legs, my arms, almost like I was taking a mini shower. It's those little things in foreign cultures that really make you appreciate the differences that we have. America may be advanced in many ways but there are certain everyday things that we seem to miss out on… Like the ability to treat ourselves to a half shower in any public bathroom.

When we headed over to the produce and meat section of the market we found stall after stall all selling a variety of fresh fruits, vegetables, meats, and fish. A lot of it looked as though it was cleaned out, the fish and meat stalls especially, and we soon found out that most of the shopping for ingredients was done in the mornings so only the scraps were left. But to us, everything was still vibrant, fresh and bountiful in its own way.

We tried our way at bartering with the fruits and vegetables and, using our not so great hand gestures we managed to get a nice bag of fresh fruit and vegetables together. One thing that made shopping at the market easy was that we would pick out everything that we wanted, then we would give it to the person working the stall and they would show us a calculator with the amount of money that we owed.

Knowing that we could buy all the fresh fruit and vegetables that we wanted, all which were incredibly cheap, made this experience more exciting. Eating out could be a little nerve wracking at times, trying my best to communicate with someone I could not really communicate with, relying solely on my intuition and allergy cards. But as I stood there picking out the freshest vegetables that I had ever seen, I began to settle into myself again and started to feel like this experience, hormones out of whack or not, was going to be a truly special one after all.

We walked the food back home, through the main park in Saigon, and on our way back we decided to stop off in an area where we saw a bunch of locals doing funny looking work outs on odd contraptions. Each one of them was on a different machine that was meant to move in a different direction, round and around, up and down, it all looked so exciting that we had to get on and give it a try even if we weren't dressed for the occasion. Getting to move our bodies, stretch out and get a little work out in, even with the sun beating down on us, was a nice way to really kick start our metabolisms to help digest that food and give us a little energy boost.

After our little "work out" we ran into some Vietnamese students who were more than happy to help us translate some different dishes and point us in the right direction of places we could go to eat great food. They were very eager to chat with us and we quickly realized that, as students, getting to speak English was very exciting and valuable for them. The taught us some words, we taught them some words and then parted ways to get back to our room.

Tip: Eat Small Meals and Shake What You Got

When traveling to a place known for having some of the best food in the world it's important to pace yourself, eating what you want, trying everything you can, but not going overboard. Sampling small dishes, snacking on fruit throughout the day is a great way to keep your body nourished without filling it to the brim and draining your energy. Walking, stretching and moving around, especially after a meal is also a great way to aid digestion.

Chapter 7:
The Quest for a Gas Burner

As much as I love eating raw foods I knew that this trip wouldn't be as exciting unless I could have the opportunity to eat some hot meals as well but after deciding that Airbnb wasn't a good option in Vietnam, we had to figure out a way to cook in our hotel room. We brought a small non-stick pan with us but we had no heating source.

Initially when we were packing we had toyed around with bringing our small electric burner, which would have been a good little backup to have as a heat source but we decided to take our chances and see if we could find a portable gas burner instead.

I am not going to pretend for a second that everyone who travels is just going to want to go out and buy a burner to cook all their meals. In fact, most won't. However, if you are truly sensitive like I am, you must be willing to put in the extra effort if you expect to eat more than raw fruits and vegetables, both of which are great and all, but eating raw vegetables can lead to a lot of gas. Again, there are other options, such as staying at a Hostel with a kitchen or renting something on Airbnb but I guess we wanted to add an extra layer of challenge.

When dining out in Vietnam eating raw food is not always the safest granted that the food is washed with untreated water sources. There was nothing more upsetting when we got a fresh salad for a meal that was clearly washed in water and we just had to sit there and watch it go to waste. Boiling water and cooking food is the only way to kill the bacteria so that it's safe for consumption. If you are cooking your own food from the markets and eating things raw and fresh you either must peel the outside layer off, like in the case of a carrot, or you have to wash it with bottled water. Seems annoying perhaps but it was quite easy.

Day one was about exploring and taking in our surroundings but by the second day we were ready to start cooking so we did a bit of research and found the name of a kitchen store that seemed like it might sell gas burners. With that information, we packed a small day bag and headed out into the depths of Saigon.

At this point we had been in Vietnam only one full day and we had stayed mostly just in the tourist area so heading out beyond was an exciting venture. It also meant that I was bringing extra's (food, bottled water, gluten free bars, dried fruits and nuts in case the rural areas didn't have anything that was safe). Sometimes I hate having to prepare stuff ahead of time, but in this type of situation you want to be safe and prepared. Carrying food can be heavy so I tend to make little snack bags of nuts and other things portioned out so that I can distribute the weight in my bag, it also makes it easier to snack.

We were prepared to venture out into the unknown, well beyond the touristy backpacking area of Ho Chi Minh. We had little to no knowledge of what was out there, beyond District 1, the main district in this major city.

Vietnam is a fairly small country, thin and long, it ranges from the North up where the capital Hanoi is, to the Central area where another major, though less touristy city resides, DaNang, and then the South where Saigon, or Ho Chi Minh, sits.

Ho Chi Minh is more of a modern city, at least in the area that we were, but we didn't know much about what to look for outside of District 1. All we knew was that we had the name of a kitchen supply store and that sometimes just setting a destination point can lead to a great journey.

On our way to find the burner we walked by an awesome outdoor market located two blocks from our hotel that was filled with fresh produce, meat, fish, and other various types of food stands. I noted how funny it was because the day before we asked the hotel for any suggestions for markets to buy food and they mentioned Ben Thanh as the only market in the area as well as a few small convenience stores. It dawned on me that when tourists ask for markets they are typically seeking the main attraction markets and chain grocery stores as no tourists ever really go shopping for groceries in the local markets, but that was exactly what we wanted to do.

We weren't ready to buy any food just yet but we saw that they had a juice stand and I started jumping with joy. I was feeling much better after getting a good night's sleep and though my hormones were still up and down, the pure excitement and curiosity I felt would momentarily put me in a good head space.

Juice is something that is safe, (just make sure you get things that are fresh and peeled) and something that I can have on the street. It almost made me feel normal, not that fresh juice is all that exciting and exotic, but this was extremely refreshing for me. For a second I thought worst case scenario while traveling if we couldn't find anything safe to eat, I could drink my weight in juice. After all, I have done my fair share of juice fasts and while I wasn't planning on doing one here, I would happily drink as much juice as I could. Best part? $1 for a whole fresh juice! And

I'm not talking the rip-me-off-Manhattan sizes, no, this was like the trucker 7/11 deluxe size juice.

As we stood in line waiting to order a fresh juice we noticed a young Vietnamese couple who appeared to be students (maybe 20 years old or so). They seemed friendly so we decided to say hello and see if they recommended anything specific that we should order, though I secretly hoping they might help us in case we ran into any language barriers with the juice lady.

We struck up a conversation with them, they spoke English quite well and luckily for us they ended up helping us order exactly what we wanted as we did have a little trouble communicating with the woman working the stand. For $2 we got two fresh juices with carrots, mango, pineapple, beets, lemon, pomelo, ginger and no ice. The young couple were super friendly and nice, they even offered to show us around if we had any questions about food or just wanted some guides as friends. We told them where we wanted to go, pointing to an area on our map and they said it was too far to walk. Little did we know at the time but Vietnamese people don't really like to walk very far, they prefer motorbikes, but for us, coming from the city we had no problem walking miles even if they thought it was a long distance.

They gave us their contact information, a few food suggestions for vegetarian, and gluten free spots, and then they hopped on their cute little motorbike and in seconds disappeared into the swarm of motorbikes.

While Vietnam, we were told, wasn't specifically considered a very warm and open country, there were a lot of friendly locals, all eager and excited to help us in any way that they could, all we had to do was ask. Sometimes just taking that chance and sparking up a conversation is usually a great way to make a new friend and get some insider information.

I'm a simple person to please, give me some fresh juice and throw me in a conversation with a nice new person and I'm happy as a clam. But I was worried about Josh, he was taking on the bulk of the planning for the trip on top of taking care of me and coaching me through my fluctuating emotions. I could tell it was a lot for him. But as we walked around I noticed that Josh was starting to feel a little relieved, sure it was overwhelming at times, it was hot and there was thousands of people everywhere but getting the juice and meeting some new Vietnamese friends was a win for us!

Tip for Helping with Translations
When trying to order or buy food, don't hesitate to ask a local for some help, especially someone who seems friendly. Maybe they are young and in school, or maybe they just have a smile on their face, either way there is no harm in asking for help. Often you will find that someone, students are more than willing to help you out, especially if it means a chance for them to practice speaking English.

With map and juice in hand we set out to find what we hoped would be the perfect kitchen appliance store to buy a gas burner. On the way, there we passed by a huge electronic store that happened to have a small gas burner out front that was affordable but we were determined to find our kitchen appliance store. It was, however, good to know that worst case we could come back here and buy one from them.

As we ventured further out we saw less and less tourists and we started to feel more and more out of place. Josh and I started to notice that we were getting some looks, we felt a little uncomfortable. Having come from a very touristy area where we were already starting to get just slightly annoyed with the random local chatters coming our way from every direction; "yes hello, American? I give you ride? You eat here? Buy from me?" we really felt a huge shift.

But out here with not a tourist in sight I quickly went from feeling comfortable to an immediate sense of unease and isolation. Was this journey a mistake? Was it really best to keep to the busy tourist areas? A normal fear I am sure but as we walked on we realized that while we looked out of place, no one really cared. Everyone around us was far too busy to be concerned with us. The locals were zipping along on their motorbikes or quickly pacing on foot going about their daily business, they had no time to relax other than for a quick bowl of soup.

And boy, did they eat fast. I have always been so excited about Vietnamese cuisine, the dedication, the love, the appreciation, the appreciation and skill of the food. There is something so incredibly balanced and special about Vietnamese cuisine, but what I was most surprised about was to see how quickly the average person slurped up food. I don't know why but I always imagined that the people of Vietnam all sat down to eat a beautiful meal, slowly savoring each bite. Silly, I know, but hey, I have so much more to learn.

The first few days were a little daunting, we had just arrived in a foreign country, we didn't speak the language and we didn't have any sort of cell phone or communication device. We were fully disconnected from the internet and the rest of the world around us. Though I felt electronically naked, it was really freeing and beautiful being surrounded by the unknown, even if it was a little bit scary. Being scared means you are trying something new, it's both invigorating and necessary.

We kept walking for a while, each street featured a new experience. The streets were packed with people and we spotted new foods we had never seen before. We strolled by interesting stores that we would pop into and check out, we went into different little markets, checked out the assortment of restaurants, read menus, just to see what people were serving. The sights and smells were astonishing, each place smelled incredible in its own way.

★Tip for navigating a city★

When you check out the map, try to get a lay of the land, see how the city works. Often cities are broken into different areas, the streets may be numbered and sometimes they are laid out in grid form. By sticking to simple directions, pick one street that you can walk down, a heavily populated street, and stay on that street, making notes of different land marks if you make any turns, taking pictures of intersections if you need to. Any little thing that will keep you feeling like you have your bearings in check, will also keep your confidence up and allow you to venture into the unknown without getting too unknown.

As we walked on, I was starting to get a little bit worried that we would not find our destination, my mind started to wonder why we didn't just buy the first gas burner that we saw, and slowly I realized that I was starting to overheat a little bit. I had gone through my water, eaten my little treats and I was starting to get tired from walking around.

Josh was determined to find our market and said that we should go a little further considering we were already out there, so we kept walking. We both really like walking, we just didn't anticipate the heat or how it would affect me... I was starting to get a little grouchy from the heat, I just wanted to plop down in bed and take a swim in the air conditioning, but now, being relatively far away from our hotel, away from our little safe touristy area, there weren't too many taxi's or motorbikes in sight and I was beginning to wonder if I could even make the journey back.

All in all, that day we walked for what seemed to be a good two hours in the blistering sun until finally we found the cross street where the appliance store was supposed to be. We kept looking for the name of the kitchen store, we looked and looked, but we saw nothing, I couldn't believe it.

We tried to ask around but we got glass stares as though we were crazy, in fact most people just straight up ignored us. We weren't in tourist town anymore, this was the real heart of a Vietnamese city and the people were not quite as friendly to help us. The locals seemed much too busy to bother with two Americans walking around looking for some random store. I was starting to feel a little scared, but again Josh reminded me that all was well and that soon we'd find this place.

In that moment, we decided as a team that all hope of finding this place was lost, that it was likely that the place didn't even exist anymore. We thought that we should head back to the other store we had passed and buy the gas burner there. The beauty of an experience like this, we realized, was that the kitchen appliance store we initially seemed out was more than a destination, it was a way to take us to another part of town that we would otherwise have never seen, it forced us to venture away from the comfortable tourist area we had grown accustom to, where most people spoke English and were overly friendly in hopes of making a sale. It really took us out of our comfort zone as a couple and it really made me see how in charge we could both be in different situations and cheerlead one another on when one of us started to falter.

Once again for me it was a win because I got to see Josh in a new light as my champion and protector. I felt like even though it was brutally hot, he had my back and I was happy to see that together we came through in a big way, that we could both step up to the plate when we needed to.

I really feel like challenging situations where a couple is put into a stressful spot are good because you see where your strengths and weaknesses are. Then, having these sides come to life, you can work on resolving the problem together. Because let's face it, life will always present you with challenges, it's not about avoiding them or hoping that they won't happen, but about learning and growing yourself and as a couple.

The choice to spend your life with someone is a freaking big one! To really know if that person is the right one you have to know that they will have your back, that they will look out for you when you really need it. Taking our little journey into a very off grid part of a foreign country where we didn't speak the local language, though it was a little frightening at the time, ended up serving as a great example of how we can work together. I am so grateful beyond words as I look back knowing that we did it together and that it all turned out perfectly.

When we started to head back I was getting hungry so it was a great little surprise when I noticed out of the corner of my eye, an old man with a motorbike that had a huge sort of box on it, he was driving around selling what looked like steamed yam's and nothing else. Josh and I looked at each other with a great excitement. We showed him our translation card and he gave us the signal that it was safe (a thumbs up and smile) so we bought a few yams. For some reason, we didn't really expect it to be all that satisfying of a treat but we didn't care, we were both hungry and it was safe for me to eat.

We found a little spot on the street to sit and started to peel away the skin, something that I feel is important to do just to be safe, in case anything did touch the skin. I always keep napkins in my bag just in case, and since we didn't have a way to wash our hands, using a napkin to eat and touch the food with instead of our fingers is a good way to avoid any issues with germs.

I guess this is the part where I should mention that I'm also a germ-a-phoebe, especially when I travel but hey, I never get sick so it works for me. Josh, on the other hand, might as well not believe in germs because he sure likes to eat as though he never has a care in the world, whether we are at a fine dining restaurant in New York or eating a small bowl of unidentified soup in Vietnam. Trusting him and knowing that he would be okay every time we sat down to eat something off the street would take some adjusting for sure.

As we sat on the sidewalk in pure bliss, munching away on our treat, we were overcome with an intoxicating sweetness of the steamed yam, we may have been hungry for something more but I swear this was next level yam! With every bite, it was tender, sweet, moist and beyond satisfying. I never imagined myself just getting all lovely on a yam but Vietnam will do that to you. It was quite romantic (especially for being in a city that had little romance), watching all the bikes whizz by us. It felt good to sit together and share a small bite, and while Josh had his eye on the Banh Ii cart a block down, the yams were so filling we decided to wait to find something else on our journey back.

On our way home, we noticed a Burger King on a busy street corner filled with locals. This was a little confusing... Burger King jam packed?! Out of curiosity Josh walked in to see what it was like and noticed that the prices, compared to the local cuisine, were crazy expensive. Unlike in the states where fast food is the cheap option, it seemed that fast food in Vietnam was actually a more expensive option for food. Not only that, but it looked like the spot to be for youngsters and we had no idea for the life of us why.

We walked home, being careful to stick to streets that we recognized, though there was still much to see, and we started to get hungry again from all the smells of street food wafting into our noses. So, we started playing the *"does this restaurant look safe?"* game with each passing block.

We came across a restaurant that seemed to be a good blend of local cuisine and tourist friendly. We decided to give our allergy cards another go and see what sort of reaction the staff would have. As we started to walk around we noticed that the restaurant seemed modernized and as much as we would have loved to have more of an authentic experience, we felt safe there considering the wait staff spoke good English and the allergy cards were well received. When we showed one of the waiters the cards, he was happy to suggest some menu options that were good for me to eat. I knew that I would be limited in options but that only makes my choice easier. After all, life is like a box of vegan chocolates, you never know what you are going to get (and if it's going to be an amazing and well-crafted gem of a meal, or just a side of rice).

★Dining Out Tip★

Trusting your gut feeling may seem scary when you aren't sure that you trust yourself but the number one most important thing when you are eating is to feel comfortable. If you have any signs of discomfort when eating, that energy will transfer into your meal and thus into you. It's a lot easier than you would imagine to feel out a situation, especially when you come prepared with your allergy cards and have done your homework. At the end of the day, you are the one in charge of your health and you have to decide whether you feel at risk or not and if that risk is worth it. I could tell you that the risk is never worth it but the truth is: Sometimes the best meals I have ever had are the ones that I wasn't sure I would be able to eat until I went in and really grilled the wait staff and made sure that my food was safe. You need to be your own advocate and never be afraid to walk away or send your food back, even after you've asked a million people whether it is safe or not.

We sat down and ordered a few things, as per the waiter's suggestion on the menu, making sure to double check with the cards, asking the manager and double checking with the kitchen while they were preparing our food. Again, I know it may seem annoying or as though you are being a burden to the wait staff and quite possibly the people you are with, but it's this fear and anxiety that will not serve you if you get sick, so start practicing now so you can overcome the notion that there is anything wrong with being extra careful. You deserve to feel safe and eat a healthy meal and if others aren't going to tolerate it or make you feel less than or like you should just eat whatever is served to you because it's not that serious, you should by no means tolerate them. This is your life, you are putting your health into their hands, and you need to feel safe and good.

It doesn't help to blame someone for being ignorant to food allergies, especially when you are traveling to a foreign country. Food allergies may be an ever-growing thing in America and other places but for a lot of countries a large bulk of the people may have never heard of them so the very idea of someone not being able to eat what they are serving is preposterous. It's not their fault if they get confused, or even a little upset, it may even be offensive to them that you would deny eating their food but that is no good reason to feel like a burden and a need to apologize for what your body can and can't have.

We ended up ordering a soup with a clear vegetable broth that was clean and delicious, I swear often the simplest meals always become my favorite. We also had a heaping portion of stir fried rice noodles with vegetables, it was so tasty and fresh. The more and more we ate out, the more I realized how different the food is in Vietnam, not only is it fresh and vibrant but every ingredient is made with great attention to detail. I could really feel the love that went into every bite.

We had only been in Vietnam for two days and it was already one of the best dining experiences for me as an allergy free traveler. The complex yet simple nature of the food was refreshing, nothing was processed, everything was so fresh, and everything was bursting with natural, bold flavor.

After we ate we were about to leave when we ran into another foreigner from New York sitting and eating alone. Ironically, he was a filmmaker, who was on a personal journey through Southeast Asia: exploring Thailand, Vietnam, Laos and Cambodia, something we found that most tourists seem to do. Hitting so many different countries in a short span of time sounded exciting and we considered doing the same but we just wanted to experience Vietnam, there was so much to offer and we only had three weeks. We chatted about where we were traveling and the foods that we hoped to try for a bit, shared some translation tips for no ice and other tidbits of information we learned to eat safely on the street and then headed out.

On our way back from lunch we stumbled upon what looked like heaven in dessert form to me. The place was filled with desserts all made from soy milk, no dairy, just delicious flavored soy milk with add-ons. We showed them the cards and they gave the thumbs up, assuring us that everything in the store was safe for me to eat. We ended up eating three small desserts. The first one was just freshly made soy milk, it was absolute heaven. The second was a red bean dessert with fresh soy milk poured over it. It was so good that we had to get a second serving after devouring the first!

And the best part was, it was so cheap and delicious! A perfectly sweet finish after a day of incredible exploration with my lover, my partner in delicious crime, and my best friend. When you have so many food allergies and have dated so many jerks in the past, ones who made me out to be some food freak who couldn't eat anything, having a supportive partner made all the difference.

Being far away from home I was reminded of the little things and how important each one of them was. I realized that the more I focused on the good things, the more the other things, like not being able to eat a Banh Mi sandwich or a big bowl of beef broth didn't matter so much (though even I can't deny having a few moments of craving such a classic local meal).

After feeling stuffed and refreshed from sitting in the air-conditioned restaurant, we headed back towards our hotel and on the way there found a massive grocery store. Not just any grocery store, but one that had not only everything we could ask for but things in which we never even thought existed. Just looking at the kitchen equipment section was overwhelming, we were blown away. They had double sided knives that had a peeler and a shredder built in and even the plastic and disposable selection seemed endless. We grabbed some small little plastic bowls that we could put condiments and small bites into, we bought a silly knife that had a peeler built into it and we continued exploring.

One of the best parts about finding a large supermarket isn't the selection of produce, oh no, we kept all produce buying to the small local markets, but it's finding the basic ingredients that one would need such as, salt, oil, vinegar, and spices.

Tip for Grocery Stores

While fresh produce at the local markets is safe, you are much more likely to find products with English translations at your large super markets. You can always ask the staff to help you find the things you need. Stock up on some of the basics, think about what you will always need such as salt and oil and how you can store it while you are traveling around. Buying Tupperware containers or plastic bags will allow you store spices and other small ingredients that you can take with you from place to place. Large commercial markets are also a great place to buy dried beans and rice, a cheap and hearty meal that is easy to make.

We tried our best not to go crazy buying everything we saw, it felt like a frenzy though. It felt like we needed everything! But we didn't, to be honest shopping in markets for us, as boring as it may sound, is one of our favorite things in the whole entire world to do. Being hard-core food lovers I guess it probably makes sense but to the outside it may seem strange that we would rather get lost exploring the isles of a random market than going to a museum. We love getting the chance to check out odd and exotic ingredients, to try new things, get a feel for what the locals eat. We get a kick out of it, it's so inspiring.

Noticing that our shopping cart was getting just a little too full, we ended up putting a good amount back as was starting to go a little crazy with gadgets and ingredients that we may or may not have needed. Josh didn't think we needed the cute mini forks and spoons, or the cute napkins… I get it, I love cute small things especially kitchen stuff, I can't help myself! After all, I'm a girl, don't judge me, I think it's in my blood or something.

We found everything we needed and more but finding paper towels was not as easy as we had expected. We noticed it was rare that any restaurants offered any sort of napkin or paper towel. I was a little out of my element as I'm half miss piggy when I eat and tend to get food on my hands, face, and god knows where else. It makes sense why they wouldn't have napkins available, it is very wasteful after all, but we were not used to it and as cute as it was to have sticky hands and bits of food left on my face to munch on later I began to wonder what bugs might try to befriend us upon smelling our leftover food stains. We did however find a big pack of baby wipes that managed to help keep my germ-a-phobia in check and they smelled quite nice too.

Tip: Baby Wipes/ Hand Wipes

Baby wipes are excellent for keeping yourself clean while in a foreign country. When we were in Vietnam it was hot, we felt like every 30 minutes we needed a shower in certain places, the wipes helped us feel refreshed when we were out and about.

Turns out that mosquitos really like sweaty people. Wiping off sweat with baby wipes keeps those pesky bugs away. In case the restaurant or stall you are eating at doesn't have any napkins, having a little pack of wipes will keep you clean, a feeling that goes a long way when you are far away from home.

Also, they are a great way to disinfect your hands before or after eating a meal especially when you don't have soap and water in site.

Okay, so we totally stocked up on baby wipes, did I mention that I'm sort of a germ-a-phoebe? This completely ended up saving our asses, no pun intended! Sometimes the bathrooms we found didn't have toilet paper, and we were able to clean ourselves anytime we wanted too, like cats, except not with our tongue…although maybe next trip I'll consider it, it might be a bit weird but I suppose it would save you a couple of bucks!

Two things that we forgot to bring with us that we went in search for at the market was a sponge and some soap, very important to help us clean up after cooking. I should mention that trying to find a simple sponge was tough! For some reason, no one could understand what we were looking for, my hand miming skills of washing dishes mid-air was not a crowd pleaser either, the workers at the market really must have thought I was mental or something!

After talking to many people, they put us on the phone with someone, they even attempted to use a translator app on the phone which was great, except it couldn't translate sponge. At this point we figured we were out of luck and did our best to say thank you and walk away. The workers there were very friendly and helpful but we came up empty handed.

We spotted the bath section and found a cute pink body sponge, thinking it couldn't be much different than a regular one and tossed it in the cart. Also, while we were fully prepared to cook extensive meals in our hotel room, we weren't exactly sure how legal it was so we wanted to make sure we left everything clean just in case of any complaints. We could have easily made sure to try and stay only in places that had kitchens, and for that matter you can do the same, but we thought it would be fun to explore all the different options, and hotels in Vietnam were very affordable.

On our way back home we went back to the original appliance store that we walked past in the beginning of our journey and we bought the gas burner with 3 extra tanks of gas. Everything only cost us $15, far cheaper than it would in the states and we were really getting excited to see how much deliciously awesome food we could re-create in our soon to be hotel room turned travel kitchen.

Tip for a Portable Kitchen

If you want to be a cooking beast while traveling, consider finding a balance between bringing the absolute essentials and buying little things you can leave behind when you head out. We managed to find a miniature portable gas burner that was fairly easy to carry along but there are small and simple options that you can find online that you may want to consider bringing. Never fly with the gas canisters though! We found it was quite easy to find them in any major city that we visited, so buy a few, use them, and then get some more the next place you go. If you are traveling by bus or train, then feel free to stock up on some extras but one canister should get you a good few hours of cooking.

Our sauté pan with foldable handle was a great way to cook some basic meals and instead of bringing tongs we used some chopsticks which were great for cooking and eating. Our flexible cutting board was helpful as it barely took up any space and allowed us to cut in just about any locations. We also made good use of Tupperware for not only storing food but for eating and mixing it as well. We would use a clean Tupperware, one that was bowl shaped, make a dressing in there, toss in the food, eat some of it and then pop on the lid to store the leftovers.

Having a peeler really made life so much easier. Not only was it necessary for taking the skin off food to ensure it was safely cleaned, but it also made it easy for us to make nice salads without having to cut our food too thin. The julienne peeler that we brought was lightweight and made for a great tool to make shaved green papaya salads, a popular dish in Vietnam.

Walking out of the appliance store with burner in hand felt like a major triumph but it was hot, when we started our journey earlier that day I was wondering whether we should be walking in the heat of the day, especially being a tad bit clueless as to where we were really heading. Now, we were getting closer to our hotel but we had bought more than we realized and on top of being sweaty and tired we were wondering if we could carry it all back.

We grabbed some more water, gulped it down and pushed our way back to the hotel. After what felt like hours, but was really more like 20 minutes, we finally arrived home to our little hotel which we were determined to transform into our own small kitchen. The whole time while we were walking back we talked about what we wanted to make, what foods that we had already seen that we hoped to recreate, we were so excited to see what would come out of our little burner and non-stick pan.

Once we got back I rinsed off under the shower and before I knew it I was feeling much better, I was ready to cook, and hunger was striking again, even if it was only the hunger in my mind! Sure, we had been eating small meals throughout the day but the excitement of getting to cook in Vietnam cancelled out any rational reasons that we might consider not eating.

Bubbling with mad ideas and inspiration from the kaleidoscope of colorful street eats we'd seen from our long journey on the road that day, we were pumped to see what we could come up with. On the horizon of hunger pangs, we could see a big fat gluten free, vegan delicious, rhino-sized-dish just waiting to come into existence.

We hadn't done any major shopping, the tiny fridge in our hotel room could only hold so much but we had a good amount of vegetables to whip something up nice. The first thing we decided to make was a little sauce. In Vietnam fish sauce goes on just about everything and the most popular condiment that you will see is something called Nuoc Cham. It is basically a simple mixture of fish sauce with a little sugar, vinegar, lime, water, salt, chili and garlic. Each one various a bit with the ingredients but they are all a delicious punch to the face of umami (the taste of savory), at least that is what Josh told me.

We wanted to make our own version, I was getting jealous of seeing everyone with their fancy shmancy dipping sauce, it wasn't fair, I deserved my own dip experience gosh darn it! And though the fish sauce was certainly the obvious star in the Nuoc Cham, we figured making a sort of sweet chili garlic sauce of our own would get the job done.

Tip for Road Sauce

Something that we quickly figured out in Vietnam was how important having sauce at all times was, especially in my case. Most of the time I was eating my own hotel cooked meals, but during times when I was able to find something safe to eat it was usually quite simple, some steamed vegetables, tofu, or a basic stir fry and rice noodles, so having my own little sauce with me always added that spice in life I crave so dearly.

By taking a small water bottle or mason jar and filling it up with a homemade delicious sauce I could travel around with my own flavor blaster without risking it spilling all over and turning all my clothes into the world's biggest bug trap.

Your sauce can be made up of anything that you desire; fresh herbs, honey, sugar, ginger, garlic, chilies, salt, or anything else but it's important to have a good vinegar base as it will help preserve anything else in the sauce and kill off any possible germs. It is still important to keep it in the fridge when you can but taking it out on little journeys throughout the day is no problem at all.

Before we got to cooking we set out everything we wanted to cook with; peelers, pan, chopsticks, knife, cutting board (just like Dexter laid out his tools), only we would be working our skills on some veggie victims! We wanted to make the sauce first because it felt like the mother of all the other food we would be consuming. Josh had eaten a lot of it already and I had smelled it way too many times to not want some in my mouth, pronto!

We laid out the garlic, chilies, vinegar, honey, spices and ginger. We had found a red ginger that I had never seen before so of course we grabbed it, and boy was it intense! We later found out that red ginger is pretty much only used to marinate dog meat, eww!! But the good news - it was a great way to add kick to our sauce!

Our version of Nouc Cham would consist of vinegar, minced garlic and chili, honey, lime juice, salt, some red ginger and some water. After everything was prepped out I started to use my hand like a funnel for getting ingredients into the water bottle to make our road sauce, we didn't have anything else and it seemed like the natural thing to do. Hands are really your best tools for cooking, eating and anything really. Chilies in, garlic in, red ginger in, salt in, then rice vinegar and honey. I started to shake it like I was a paint mixer at Home Depot, to try an incorporate all the ingredients into one big love liquid of spices and goodness.

As I finished up the sauce, Josh had gotten our new stove burner all set up. During this time, I hadn't realized how late it had gotten and we had gone from ravenous to a zombie like "I will eat anything right now" mode of existence. The plans switched from making some epic meal to; *What's the quickest and tastiest thing we could whip up in seconds?* Josh had already peeled

79

and sliced the vegetables, and was getting ready to toss them in the hot pan.

Let me back it up for second and set the scene. We were cooking with one tiny burner in a hotel room with windows that did not open and with just enough space to put a cutting board and a few things on the table, we didn't want to overwhelm ourselves after being in the heat all day but we wanted to make the cooking work, without alerting the hotel.

Secondly, the ingredients were so fresh we just wanted to bring out the essence of what the food really was trying to say to us. Not wanting to overcomplicate the beautiful vegetables, we ended up making a fresh stir fry, using bean sprouts in place of noodles because we hadn't bought fresh rice noodles yet. All in all, the meal was simple, delicious, fresh and just what we needed.

That night after resting from a minor food coma that ensued from gorging on our first home-hotel-cooked meal we were ready for more exploration. Armed with the words for no ice, we headed out to find a spot to get some late-night drinks, hoping to find some nice cocktails was the name of the game for our impromptu date night celebration. It might not seem like much, what with being in Vietnam and finding a little burner to cook meals on, but we like to celebrate the small victories. Why not? After all, life is one big journey and you should appreciate every day. It's like our society only wants to celebrate proper holidays, birthdays and awards, but each day can be magic.

As we explored the darkened streets, glowing with neon signs, we walked by so many crazy clubs with blaring music, strobe lights and screaming foreigners, but we didn't get pulled in by that ambiance, we wanted something a bit more chill.

Suddenly it hit us, this city is not really built for romance. True, we didn't see locals holding hands or making any sort of physical gestures to their partners in our short time in Saigon, but it wasn't until we attempted our first date night that we really felt just how unaffectionate of a city we were in, and as we later found out, how taboo it was to hold hands, or any PDA for that matter, while walking down the street and out in public.

For me, being half Ecuadorian, affection is in my blood... And I found it strange, at first when I started to feel eyes on us when I would rub Josh's back or arm, so, for the sake of not standing out, I did my best to resist the urge, I really wanted to respect the culture.

As we searched for our magical romantic bar we eventually got lured in by a staff member running a two-story bar type club not far from our hotel. They promised us two drinks for the price of one, which we later found out meant that each drink we buy we get a second for free but that we each needed to buy a drink. Did I mention we were both lightweights and typically liked to split one drink not end up with four?

We were lead up an endless flight of stairs to where they promised us a nice rooftop bar area to relax and sit at. As we walked up each flight of stairs every floor became more and more confusing. Every flight we went up sounded like a completely different landscape, from intense techno club music to trance Asian inspired electro fusion, we had no idea what we were getting into, it felt like we were in some crazy Alice in Wonderland type house.

Finally, when we got to the top balcony after about five flights of stairs, we were outside, it was peaceful and calm and it had a nice breeze. It was just like they promised, very nice and relaxing. However, literally no one else was there which we weren't sure if that was a good thing or not, but it felt nice and romantic just for the fact that we weren't surrounded by swarms of tourists and locals trying to sell us something. There was some groovy music playing and the air was fresh but when we caught our breath after walking so many flights we began to wonder why no one else was there and if we had made the right choice. After a second, trust set back in and we decided that all was as it should be.

With a renewed sense of calm and appreciation for our little date night, we started to look through the menu, it was all in English so we were set! There were so many drinks! *What we should get?* we wondered. Oddly enough none of the drinks sounded very Vietnamese, they were more of your standard drinks you'd find at any tropical resort but we didn't care much.

We both liked the sound of the Pina Colada, it was sweet and hopefully not too strong. (Did I mention we are real light weights?) So, we waved the waiter over and started to inquire if it had any dairy at all or any gluten in it. We showed him my allergy free cards and said asked for nice ice even though we realized that the drinks wouldn't be as refreshing as they would be with ice, it was better to be safe than sorry…

After we ordered our drink, which turned out to be two drinks not one, we had a great idea to order some ice on the side so we could see if it was safe. Moments later we asked for cups of ice and were pleasantly delighted that it was the cylinder ice from the factories, big score for us! I cannot begin to say how nice it is to have an iced drink hit your hot parched lips when you are in a tropical climate… It's pure ecstasy!

Thankful that the drinks weren't too strong we somehow managed to finish them, we left the second two drinks a little less consumed as we started to feel the effects and became quite sleepy. We were super tired from the day of journeying and walking around in the heat so we walked home a little tossed and passed out hard the second our heads hit our pillows.

⋆Tip for Drinking⋆

Even though we aren't big drinkers, I know that it's a fun thing to do during any trip and with prices so cheap you can really get ahead of yourself with the drinking, but it's important to be careful. It might suck to have to hold off on ice for a refreshing cocktail, even though the asking for ice on the side really did save us on many occasions, but it's an important one to remember.

Also, it gets really hot in Vietnam so be sure to drink lots of water, especially while you are drinking alcohol. For every glass of booze you drink, make sure you drink at least a glass of water, the last thing you want to do is be seriously hungover in such intense heat. It's one thing to feel the effects of alcohol the next day after a late night of drinking when you are in the comforts of your own home, but it's another in a developing country in the dead of summer, it can really put a damper on your trip, so be careful out there and stay hydrated.

Chapter 8:

Getting Down with the Locals

Josh being the epic YouTuber that he is, posted a video to his channel asking if any of his fans lived in Vietnam and might want to show us around. I hadn't considered the idea but I was really glad that he did, what a way to see the real heart of the country. We both knew that meeting and spending time with locals would only add to our experience and so when we found out that a few people had reached out to us we got really excited to see what might come of it.

On our final day in Saigon before we had planned to head out to the Mekong Delta, we met up with a fan of his named Kelly. We knew absolutely nothing about her but we were really excited to see where we might end up. We had hoped to do some filming in the local market followed by a little cooking segment and she gratefully agreed to show us around and be our translator. She also said she had a great place for us to cook and was happy to help us in any way that we needed. Wow, our own personal guide who was excited and into food, what more could we ask for?

When Kelly pulled up to our hotel she was with her cousin and they were on a motorbike, something we had been interested in but hadn't had the chance to try. They looked a little bit like death traps from the way people drove here, but we were open to it.

Kelly was very nice but quite shy at first. She was about 17 years old, had a simple and polite smile and was very friendly and warm. She was incredibly sweet and adorable. She was inquisitive, intelligent and spoke good English. Her cousin was also very friendly but it was clear that he didn't speak English as well as Kelly and the two of them mostly joked between themselves.

After we chatted for a few minutes they took us to the local market and Kelly started showing us around, going from stand to stand as we looked on with wide eyes. The sheer amount of new vegetables that we had never seen before was astounding! Josh and I felt like little kids with a grown up around "What's that? And that, what's that? And that?"

We were pointing at everything. Kelly was so sweet and fun, she was patient with us translating pretty much everything we pointed to, though some of the things we saw had no proper English translation. We just wanted to absorb and learn everything that was there, we couldn't help ourselves. We had spent days wondering what these ingredients were and we were curious how they could be used for cooking, she was knowledgeable.

The market, already a chaotic place, only got more chaotic as Josh did his best to capture everything on the camera while I kept saying "And this, what is that? And that, what is that? That? This?" Kelly, being the perfect, sweet and knowledgeable host was keeping up. I loved it! She even shot us a little humor when I had finally asked so many times "What can we do with this?" she finally said "Cook it and eat it."

To say that Kelly was a real sport and extremely helpful would be an understatement, she was a food angel! She must have thought we were crazy about food (we are). There was a lot of stuff that we could recognize at the market, fresh produce that we had used in the states, but there were so many more ingredients that we had never seen before. Green spiked cucumber cactus looking things, long strands of purple rope like vegetables that almost looked like shoestring onions, turns out they were actually shredded banana blossoms. I can't get over how freaking delicious they were! Raw, cooked or tossed in anything for garnish, it was pure genius! The whole experience of being there brought me back to my childhood; going to local markets in Ecuador, bustling with food vendors, vegetable purveyors, and people laughing, drinking and dancing around.

We sort of went a little nuts buying food, we couldn't help ourselves. We bought some of what we did recognize just because it was familiar and we knew we'd like it, and we bought even more of the things we had never seen before, just to find a good balance of adventure and comfort.

With six bags packed with all sorts of exotic goodies we headed back to the hotel, packed a few things, grabbed some water and we were out again. Kelly had invited us to hang out and cook at her uncle's house. She had arranged for us to follow her and her cousin on motorbikes. Motorbikes! This was our chance to see what it felt like being inches away from cars whizzing past the world, praying not to get squashed like a fly on the windshield of a vehicle.

First off getting on a bike with someone you don't know is already something to think about. As soon we got on, I wasn't even fully seated and we were already jetting off into traffic... Shit! My heart started racing with adrenaline and fear, I was terrified of roller coasters and this felt a lot like that but somehow way scarier. After all, roller coasters had a track and a direct path, these things had a mind of their own. After a few minutes of being on the road and seeing Josh in front of me turning back to check on me, smiling and laughing, I felt a wash of calm and laughter come over me, this was fun and crazy as all hell!

The wind blowing in my face as we rushed by the city streets, doing our best to weave in and out of traffic, never going too fast but never really knowing which direction that the bike would go to avoid any oncoming traffic. There was a flow involved in all the drivers, it was like they were in the matrix or something, there was no fear in anyone's face so it made it much easier to keep calm. I swear it was like a scene out of a movie, there were hardly any lights, not much in terms of rules of the road, it was all this beautiful yet chaotic orchestra.

The truth is, we didn't know whether our drivers were fully aware of their surroundings or not but it felt better to think that they did. The drivers seemed to know just where to go, weaving between two big trucks here, flying in the middle of the intersection and just missing the old lady there, it was all a big game to them as they seemed to avoid life defying accidents moment to moment. I started to relax, this was their life and I was just a viewer taking it in. I reminded myself repeatedly "Jaquy you are totally fine!" With that new perspective in mind, the beauty of Ho Chi Minh took my breath away, its diversity and beauty were sensational.

As we drove on the motorbikes, taking in all the scenery, getting to see a variety of districts, getting deeper and deeper into the city, I began to realize that where we were headed was a place few foreigners had ever ventured too before. There was a divine trust in me that wherever it was that we were going, even if we had only known Kelly and her cousin for an hour or so, was perfectly right.

Motorbike Tips

As we would come to find out, Motorbikes, not Taxis, were the best way to travel around within a city. Taxis were great for long distance but motorbikes were cheap and easy to catch on just about every corner in Saigon. Even though it may seem scary at first, they are very safe, the drivers really do know what they are doing, it's just that when you are not used to being on a bike it can seem a little scary at first.

Most of the drivers however did not speak good, if any, English, so having the name of where you are going printed clearly on paper or on a phone is very helpful. Most hotels are happy to call you a motorbike and help you get exactly where you are going.

When we arrived at her uncle's place a small dog in the street was barking at us and the people around were staring, it was obvious that we were the only foreigners around, but we just smiled, waved and they waved back.

As we walked up to her uncle's house we saw motorbikes everywhere. He had a large garage door leading inside to his kitchen and all lined up along the sides of the walls were motorbikes, there must have been 15 of them. Kelly's uncle, as it turns out, was asleep, which at first seemed a little odd until we learned that it was common to work in the morning, eat, rest for a bit, and get back to work. It reminded me more and more of growing up in Ecuador; waking up early, working, coming home for lunch, taking a siesta then heading back to work in the afternoon. It's crazy how so many cultures are so similar in some ways, and completely different in other ways… While in America we seldom do this, because it gets so hot during the day, taking a mid-day rest makes a lot of sense.

Kelly's Uncle's kitchen was nice, it had a gas stove with an oven (which as it turns out was quite rare), big open space, lots of room, and natural light coming in from the outside. This was a huge step up for us from our make-shift hotel kitchen, to have counter space to play around with, a proper stove…, this was a different animal and we knew we could churn out some killer food for everyone.

New space to cook, new ingredients we'd never used, it was like being on the Food Network show Chopped again! Except this time, I had no blue hair and Josh wasn't competing against his brother, no, we were both competing simply with time as hunger was setting in pretty hard. It's always funny being in a stranger's kitchen, especially one you have yet to meet, at first I felt a little uncomfortable moving their stuff, without knowing them and gauging their vibe, I couldn't be sure of how strict or laid back they were.

I found myself opening every drawer and feeling a bit like a thief looking to see what goodies they had to play with while doing my best to be respectful. It is after all, someone else's home and we were guests, we didn't know their rules, or much of the culture's rules for that matter. Kelly put us at ease when she just said use whatever we felt like just as long as we put it away and leave it as it was found. We immediately felt relaxed when Kelly made it clear that we could play and use whatever inspired us and that her uncle was more than happy to have us.

Before I started to prepare anything, I took out my red foldable cutting board, chopsticks and vinegar, and Kelly started to chuckle. "What's that for?" she asked.

"Well, I have Celiac disease and multiple food allergies, and this red 'Ferrari' cutting board allows me to safely cook anywhere."

"Really? Can you get sick or something if you use another cutting board?"

"Yeah, if it's wood. It's easy to get sick from cross contamination. Even the tiniest bit of wheat having touched a cutting board can make me sick."

"Oh wow… So, you are gluten free then?"

"Yeah!"

"Oh cool!"

To our great surprise, Kelly not only knew what it meant to be gluten free but she had done some gluten free baking and was quite into it. It was like we had hit the lottery, she was very health conscious, ate mostly vegetarian even, wow, out of all the people in Vietnam who knew nothing about food allergies, we had found one of the few that apparently knew quite a lot.

We started chopping away and teaching Kelly and her cousin some tricks we knew about cooking various vegetables; cutting, chopping, mincing, and sautéing everything we bought to create a large feast. Midway through cooking, her uncle's daughter, a tiny little girl around the age of four, came down to the kitchen from her mid-day nap, she was absolutely adorable. She wanted to play so I carefully started to show her how to use a knife and side by side she and I were cutting veggies, it was so much fun!

As we started to wrap things up and get ready to eat we found out that Kelly's cousins didn't really eat vegetables. At first, we were a little confused but the more we begun to understand the Vietnamese culture, the more sense it made, for they are a very meat heavy culture. Had we known this earlier, we would have gladly bought some meat for him to eat, we were simply to consumed by all the magic at the market to think to ask. s

We were hoping that part of his distaste for vegetables came from his lack of trying them and that by getting him involved, and showing them him how to cook, that he would at least give the vegetables a try but he didn't seem very interested even if it did smell and look wonderful. Luckily, we had bought some clam like creatures that we steamed with a fresh made tamarind sauce that he happily munched on.

To our surprise, it was Kelly who really loved vegetables, so much so that she was vegetarian. We didn't know that she was vegetarian before we met her but the more we found out about her, the more our minds were blown. It may not seem like much but if you knew much about Vietnamese food culture as we were starting to, you'd realize that she was a unique anomaly. Out of all the Vietnamese people we could have had this experience with, it was truly amazing that we met her, it felt like divine food intervention.

Not only was she one of the first people who didn't scoff that I was vegan, she was quite over the moon that I was! She said on occasion she would have to eat meat, after all she was 17, living in South East Asia, and had parents who were insistent that meat was important for her to grow and be strong. But while her parents fed her meat whenever they could, she preferred vegetables and was truly the odd one out, being a vegetable lover in a meat-centric culture that even served chicken for breakfast (and sometimes meat inspired desserts).

When we asked her why she seemed to have a better understanding of Western Culture and a closer connection to it than most of her friends, she attributed it to watching YouTube cooking channels and expanding her knowledge of food and health through the internet. Her friends actually referred to her as the "Hippie" of the group, a funny concept to me, as she looked nothing like the hippies that I have come to know in NY, but I suppose a Vietnamese person that is practically vegan, loves to bake, and has a unique view of her culture, could be seen as a hippie where she comes from. She may have not had dreadlocks or smell of hemp, but I suppose she was the embodiment of a hippie in her own way (had the 60's counterculture started in Vietnam).

I love how the information accessible online can inspire and connect people from around the world in the most unpredictable of ways, it's explosive and so exciting to see how knowledge can freely spread, especially to countries that have been based on tradition for so many years. Her view of eating fresh food, eating well, having balance in life, making food from other cultures, it was all influenced from around the world. How freaking epic is that! I know it sounds obvious today but when you really think about how new the internet is, it's quite a special thing. Sometimes it takes going to another country, one far different than yours, to really see how powerful certain mediums, like YouTube, can be to open up our world to the ways of other cultures.

Kelly, being one of the few in her friend group who had been exploring the world around her through the internet, had really learned so much about food and loved baking. Kelly told us that it was uncommon for a traditional Vietnamese house to have an oven, which we later found out was true for most of the country. I can't imagine what cooking back home would be like if I didn't have an oven, roasting veggies, baking yummy gluten free treats, what would I do? As I thought about it I realized the next few weeks would be a test to see what it was like.

Being intense lovers of the Vietnamese food culture, we were both really intrigued to learn about why people in Vietnam loved food so much. Their food is filled with flavor, skill, attention to detail and cooked with great passion, unlike a lot of the food that many Americans eat every day. When we brought this up with

Kelly she seemed a little confused, from her perspective she saw things quite differently.

Kelly told us that for the average person food wasn't much more than fuel, most of the workers simply ate as much and as fast as they could to keep a full belly, believing it would give them good energy for the day. To them it wasn't about sitting down and simply appreciating food, sure the flavors were incredibly delicious, but it was what they were used to eating and for a lot of Vietnamese people they believed that they needed to eat to keep their energy up, not so much because they were savoring the dish.

Kelly said that if we started to watch the locals eating that we would probably start to notice how quick they ate. This was still a shock to us but it did kind of make sense the more that we thought about it. I'm sure this was a bit of a generalization as obviously, there is a craft to the food and people must appreciate the variety of dishes, but I suppose what is foreign to us, what seems and tastes exotic, is really just everyday food for someone else. In America, we are exposed to so many different cuisines, and have access to very authentic takes on other cultures food, but that isn't how it is in Vietnam. YouTube may be exposing people like Kelly to new styles and ways of enjoying food, but it hasn't spread much in the country yet.

One thing I noticed that I always found interesting was how little the people cooking the food cared about praise for their delicious meals. In America, it has become all about glamorizing chefs, making them feel special, giving restaurant reviews, sharing our opinions about the food and judging their creations on cooking competitions. But in Vietnam they really didn't care what you thought of their food, they just wanted you to eat. And for good reason, for one they probably already know that their food is amazing and for another, they had been likely making a select few dishes for very many years, following recipes that have been passed down from generation to generation, recipes that were tried and proven in their deliciousness.

Talking about food with Kelly was really eye opening but I was getting hungry. Finally, it was time to eat! We put all the food in bowls at the table and began passing each dish around, family style. Kelly's cousins mostly ate the shellfish that we cooked in the sweet tamarind sauce, it smelled so good, even if I couldn't try it, and the rest of us began chomping down on the veggies, they were incredibly fresh and delicious.

I know most vegans can't stand the smell or site of animal foods but that's just not me. I like and enjoy other people eating what they like and am always happy to see Josh eating meat even if I can't stand the taste anymore. I do love animals but I am not a Vegan who speaks out for animal rights or yells at people who don't follow the same diet as I do. I believe that everyone should have a choice in what they eat and while I think that you can be completely happy and satisfied from living on a Vegan diet, I know some people need their animal proteins and respect that.

Meat or not, we had so many vegetable dishes coupled with a few mini salads and sauces that I was in food heaven. Somehow, we managed to finish eating pretty much everything. It was a feast that could have fed six hungry grown men, and we devoured it!

As we were finishing up and getting ready to head back home Kelly asked if we'd like to try some traditional desserts. How could we say no? I may have been stuffed but that doesn't mean I didn't have space for dessert! Josh and I have a sort of unspoken rule that every meal should end with a dessert. It doesn't matter how full we are, we just take a few breaths, maybe stretch the stomach a little and go right after it, even if it's just a few bites of something sweet to clean our mouth out and end the meal.

As we jumped back onto the back of some new motorbikes being driven by two men who were friend of Kelly's Uncle, I started to feel like James Bond on a top-secret mission. Kelly wanted to take us deep into the heart of Chinatown, a place I hadn't even realized existed in a country so close to China. Upon hearing this, we were thrilled, let me just preface this statement with the fact that if you suggest going to Chinatown in any part of the world to Josh or I we jump for joy like little kids going to a candy shop.

As we zipped through traffic we both kept looking at each other smiling like giddy kids headed to Disneyland. Were we nerds? Hell yea! And we loved every second of it. The crazy part is as intense and crowded as the streets were in the main tourist district of Vietnam, this was so much more intense, there were more people on the road and their driving seemed even more reckless yet controlled.

When we pulled up to a small, unassuming stand, we had another taste of being the only foreigners for what felt like miles, getting stares in every direction, but this time we had the added bonus of being guided by a local, the secret key to the heart of the city. It was hot, we were coming from a long and tiring day but we were determined to try something new, something that only a local would eat.

We were both glad that we were there with Kelly, it felt safer somehow, being there with someone who spoke the language and looked relaxed, it put us at ease. With her translation skills, any fear I had of being poisoned by gluten went away. Still the translation part was interesting to me because doing that in a touristy area where other foreign travelers probably asked similar questions is one thing, but out here in the more untapped parts was a completely different experience.

The lady that Kelly spoke to had a small metal cart filled with a variety of different ingredients on the side of a busy street. There were little plastic seats and tables next to her cart which Kelly told us to sit in. The woman had a bunch of large metal bowls, each filled with something different, everything ranging from what looked like bubble tea tapioca, to yellow sludge with little specks of yellow dots in it, to black pudding, to other things that looked like they had been made in the creepy crawler machine, or perhaps were still creeping around in there - it was honestly hard to tell. Besides one thing that appeared to be maybe tapioca pearls, pretty much everything was completely unrecognizable, we didn't care much about what it was so long as it was gluten free, vegan and safe for me to eat. Everything looks so odd but we were excited to give them a try! Why not right?

Kelly pretty much ordered for us now that she had a good idea what our preferences were. As we waited for our desserts to arrive, Kelly began to tell us about this famous little spot we were about to eat at, and its national prized dessert called Che. It was also one of Kelly's favorite dessert so this really did feel like a special ending to our adventurous day of markets, cooking in stranger's homes and learning more about the local culture.

Che, which you simply must try if you stumble upon it, is made up of a variety of different sweets, jellies, lotus seeds, lychee, grass jelly (safe for those with celiac disease), a whole bunch of different flavors and textures, usually mixed with crushed ice (which she assured us was safe) and sometimes it was even topped with coconut milk. They even had split mung bean jelly which was odd until we tried it and were blown away by how well the beans took to sweet, as every jelly was sweet in its own way.

Even for Kelly it was so hard to pick out just one dessert so we ended up getting six small desserts total between the three of us, when in Ho Chi Minh, right? I was able to have one of them because we knew that it was safe for sure, so that was important and great for me! You get to choose a topping and so we chose fresh coconut milk and shaved ice.

When we got our order, we took a few moments to capture some pictures and then I quickly began to dig in. I really was skeptical of that yellow mung bean dessert, it looked kind of like slime with beans and coconut milk, not appealing I know, but the second I started tasting it I was hooked hard core. Holy amazeballs, it was so oddly delicious.

I had never had anything like it before. It was slimy in a good way, it had hints of memories of exotic drinks and desserts that I'd had back home in Chinatown, New York. But let's just say that the most exotic dessert I'd ever had back home in Chinatown was a mild version of the most basic dessert in Vietnam. Josh and I were immediately hooked! One of the desserts that Josh was munching on looked even crazier than the one I had, it had about 6 different layers of jellies, lychee, and other unidentified toppings. There was a moment where I wish I could have taken a bite but he did a great job explaining the flavors to me and I felt like I was right there in his little mouth eating away with him.

While we sat, and stuffed our faces with Che we started talking about the perception of beauty in Vietnam and Kelly gave us some unique insight into why we were getting stares by some of the locals in this area, which was not, apparently, for the same reason that we assumed.

According to her, to the locals, we looked like gods. What? Gods, uhh… me? Thanks, but yeah don't think so! But really, it's the truth. According to their culture, the way that we look; our wide eyes, button like noses, creamy white skin, we are considered to be their perfect ideal image of beauty and believe it or not she told us that a lot of Vietnamese people go to great lengths to try and obtain a similar image.

There are women who dye their skin white and change the color of their eyes and hair to appear to be more white. Although I'd experienced something a bit like this in China and Japan when traveling somehow, I didn't think of it in Vietnam. She began to tell us that in the past it was different, woman used to chew some special leaf to dye their teeth black because it used to be thought that having black teeth made a woman beautiful and attractive. It was interesting seeing as how we had noticed a few older women in that area with almost black teeth who, I at first believed to have poor hygiene. It's amazing how far information can go beyond assumption.

This was super interesting to me because it just reminded me of how different cultures perceive beauty and the lengths one will go to obtain what they think it to be. To think about how many people are trying to look like the standard for models that they see on TV and in magazines, even if they know fair well that it's only through the magic of Photoshop that the models end up looking so perfectly skinny and super tan. So here we are with all this pressure coming from both sides, everyone wanting to look like someone else and yet so few truly appreciating their own inner and outer beauty. Food for thought. And speaking of food…

After we finished chomping away at our weird and delicious Che treat, Kelly took us for a walk towards a pagoda. On the way, there we noticed lots of street vendors and we decided to stop at a vendor who was selling some street donuts. Josh and I had noticed them a lot while roaming around the day before, they had this intoxicating aroma that reminded me of my childhood so I just had to know what was in them.

Just smelling it reminded me of fresh donuts from bakeries with cold milk, the old days before being diagnosed celiac when I ate a lot, and I mean A LOT, of wheat. I asked Kelly if she could translate to see if they were safe and it turns out that they were! *JACKPOT*! I thought. The lady had a whole bunch of these round, sesame covered donuts, filled with a variety of fillings like red bean and coconut. The donut itself was made from glutinous rice flour (which does not have gluten in it) and so delicious. Kelly was sweet to be thorough in asking about where she made it and what else was made in the same area. So, good news, if you see these awesome donuts, even though you should be careful because often they are made with wheat, you might be able to eat them! Banh Tieu was the name of the donuts, they aren't hard to find around the streets, just look for a lady carrying a little basket of treats and you just might be in luck.

We felt safe with Kelly there because you could tell she really cared about making sure that anything I ate was good for me to eat. And thank heaven she was there because what would have otherwise just have been eye candy for me instantly became belly love bombs. I couldn't recall the last time I could have such a decadent treat from the street, not one that looked like this at least. Still, eating anything off the street for me, and anyone, possess some bit of risk, it's always good to be thorough and mindful, but having a local with you works wonders, especially one who cares.

Tip for Exploring Street Food

Try to find a friendly local who is willing to take you out exploring. We found a few places that gave street food tours in each major city, one of them was even someone who gave an all gluten free tour, however, unfortunately for us she was away when we were there. Either way it's worth noting that there are not only locals who you can pay a small amount of money to help you navigate the street food but there are also a bunch of foreigners living in Vietnam who host their own tours and know the food really well. If you can't find a street tour, you may be able to find a friendly local standing nearby who is happy to translate for you.

When we arrived at the pagoda, a beautifully hand carved masterpiece, out front we saw a man selling pigeons. Kelly told us that for about $1 you could buy a pigeon and set it free, otherwise they would be killed as an offering to the Gods. I wondered for a moment if he would let us free them all, or if perhaps he just goes back out and catches them all after we leave? Kelly wasn't quite sure what really went on so we decided to set a few free in the hopes that they flew far away!

When we entered, the beautiful pagoda covered with statues and hand carved designs, there were incense burning near the entrance. As soon as the smell hit my nostrils I felt an immense peace and intense calmness wash over me. She brought some incense for us to burn and we went over to the main area in the pagoda to pray.

The pagoda was gorgeous, it was red and gold and the energy everywhere was radiating a love and serenity that I had not felt in a long time. I loved the feeling of being there because it reminded me of traveling with my parents through Japan. It made me miss my dad but I knew in remembering him that his spirit was there with me in that very moment.

In Vietnam, there are pagodas everywhere but they all have their own unique differences and energy to them. They seem to blend together when you see them from afar but upon entering, taking your shoes off and praying, you feel and see the differences in each sacred place. After we finished praying Kelly told us to bow 3x to withhold the tradition which we did before heading out. I wanted to stay longer to hold onto that feeling of having memories of my dad near my heart but told myself that I could come back to that moment anytime, I just had to remember.

As we were walking towards the main road to catch another motorbike back into the city the sun was starting to set and a golden light was illuminating everything around us making the night feel even more magical. While Kelly flagged us down a couple of motorbikes to take us back, we spotted another food cart that we simply couldn't take our eyes off.

There was a lady who had seven grills going, all extremely hot, flames billowing below, she was pouring a yellowish batter into the pans. We were stuffed from all of the eating that day but Kelly explained to us that this was a very special dish in Vietnam called Banh Xeo.

Banh Xeo is a dish that is made from blending up pre-soaked rice flour, usually with a little turmeric to give it a yellow color and then it is fried up in a hot pan with lots of oil and usually topped with shrimp, pork, and some other seasonings. Sometimes the batter is made with egg but luckily this one was not.

Even though Kelly made sure it was safe, ordering me one without any meat or seafood, when I really thought about it, I just couldn't put anything else into my body, I was stuffed to the brim, so we decided to take one to go, which only cost us $1. We said goodbye to Kelly, who mentioned that perhaps we could take a trip to visit her grandmother tomorrow, and then we jumped on the back of two motorbikes and we were on our way back to the hotel in a flash.

When we got back home we pulled out our little Banh Xeo treat. It came with some bean sprouts, a little of the chili fish sauce and some fresh lettuce to wrap it in. We re-cleaned the lettuce, I pulled out my own little sauce, and started to dig in. Unfortunately, because we had waited too long, the Banh Xeo wasn't fresh and crispy anymore, it had become quite soggy from the journey home and it wasn't all that tasty. Josh said he had gotten one on the first morning that I slept in and it had been fantastic. He said the freshness was so important, having a crispy pancake made all the difference. This got me thinking.

Even though the woman at the stand was happy to accommodate me, she displayed a little reluctance to alter her dish by leave out the meat and fish. It's no surprise that a lot of cooks don't want to change their dishes up. After all, they have spent many years perfecting their recipes, or have been keeping up a family tradition for a long time and the very idea of changing it means that there is a change in the flavor and it might get ruined. I can't tell you how many times I have been to restaurants where the chef insists on me not trying something because it will be "flavorless" without an ingredient such as butter. Of course, when I finally give him a pep talk and remind him that I don't even really remember what butter tastes like, he ends up making something incredibly delicious.

Having tried the Banh Xeo that sat out to long gave me all the more reason to want to learn how to make it myself, it was rice based and meat and fish aside, safe for me. The texture of the crepe like batter, when fried, seemed really crispy and beautiful.

They even had a version where they fried it into little balls that were stuffed with all kinds of goodies called Banh Khot. I hoped that somewhere along our journey we would learn the secret to this Vietnamese staple, for now, more exploring.

Chapter 9:

On Your Left, a Place Where No Outsider Has Gone Before

By the time, we had gotten home it seemed that we had made a dear friend. Kelly had casually mentioned to us as we whizzed away on our motorbikes that maybe on our way out the next day we could visit her grandmother. At the time, we didn't think much of it but were more than willing to entertain the idea I mean, come on, more locals that we could hang out with! Um yes, please! And more cooking? Double score! We had plans to leave Ho Chi Minh city the following day and head south towards the Mekong Delta by bus, after which we would fly all the way south to Hanoi out of the Mekong Delta Airport but upon checking our email when we got to the hotel we had a letter from Kelly saying that if we were interested that her father could drive the three of us to her grandmother's house, which was midway towards where we were staying the following day. We could spend the day with her grandmother on the Mekong Delta and then they would drop us off at the bus to head to our next destination. It worked out well because we had yet to book a bus ticket for our 3-hour journey to Can Thon where we would be staying on a small and cozy bungalow in a very intimate part of the jungle.

I was tired as all hell, it had been a long day and my mood was up and down. The weather was hot and my body was drained but I just had to keep on pushing, I couldn't help myself. It all sounded too much fun, a chance to meet Kelly's grandmother who she had said was an incredible cook, uh, yes please!

Before we called it a night, Josh wanted to head out into the streets, since it was our last night in Ho Chi Minh city. It was our final chance to explore the food scene a little more before we said goodbye to the bright city of lights, and mouth-watering street food. I had a blast watching Josh get excited about trying more food, although I must say I hand's a clue at this point as to where he was storing all this food. The man has a serious talent and dedication to eating, it was the damnedest and cutest thing I had ever seen! After he scarfed down some grilled chicken wings and a nice bowl of noodle soup, we packed up our things and fell fast asleep.

The next morning, we jumped into a cab with all our stuff and headed to Kelly's family's house. We met her parents who were super sweet and welcoming. Kelly, her dad, Josh and I went out to pack the car. Since I knew we'd be traveling around breakfast I already had a little protein shake that I made in our hotel room, as well as some fruit and nuts, just in case I got hungry on the road.

The three of us got into the car along with a driver that they had hired and we were off. The drive was breath-taking, we drove through open fields, rice paddies, farms, and road side stalls, straight along one road. It was so much more rural than the first few days of our journey in the city, and it felt like a breath of fresh air.

Midway through the drive we stopped to get food at what seemed to be a local rest stop. Kelly told us this was one of the more famous ones that her family had a tradition of stopping at whenever they took the trip down to see her grandmother. When we walked in, we saw a bunch of other locals sitting at big cafeteria like tables, the place was very large and the food was flying in the open kitchen behind the tables.

Expecting that the rest stop would not to have much for me to eat, I sat there patiently while everyone else ordered pork with rice. Kelly was sweet enough to get me some steamed rice and steamed vegetables so I could have a little something. She was very careful when ordering for me and even though it was a simple dish of steamed greens and rice it was amazing! They even had some chili sauce on the side that I scarfed down. American pit rest stops this was not! I had never eaten broken rice before and the texture was like a pilaf and rice pudding, it was very light and fluffy. Even at the local rest stop out towards the more rural area of Vietnam, the food was still amazing.

After our lovely meal, we drove another 45 minutes or so and as we got closer, I noticed just how different the country side and pace of life was beyond the city limits. The Mekong Delta is known for its famous floating markets and villages and we were eager to have a chance to glimpse into that life. There were organized tours but we were hoping to find a way to jump on a small boat (often called a sampan), and do some local cooking. Perhaps shop around the local market and see what local delicacies were like there.

The original plan was that when we arrived at our next destination, the homestay we had booked online where we would be spending the night, to ask the host if they could set us up with a special floating tour. We were happy to pay extra if someone would take us out on a tour of the floating markets just so we could film a little cooking segment on the water. We had done a lot of research on the floating markets, there was the big famous one called Cai Rang Market that was more for buying in bulk, this was mostly where the tourists went on their boat trips to look at the local way of life, and then there was a smaller one called Phong Dien Market where you could buy small ingredients and dishes. The smaller floating market was the one we hoped to get a glimpse of but little did we know our plans were about to take a major turn.

When we pulled up to her grandmother's house, though you could hardly call it a house, I was in total shock. Here I was thinking that we would be headed to some random little house to do a bit of casual hanging out and maybe some cooking, but when we pull up to what was more like a village with a fleet of people inside waiting for us! My mind began to run in confused excitement.

The place was breathtaking and beautiful; all open, unique architecture, handmade, mostly wood, well drafted designs, it was all just stunning. There were hammocks out front covered by a spacious wooded roof and the house overlooked the Mekong Delta river. A creek ran through their property by the cooking area, and as we got the mini tour we soon realized they were literally part of a small village. We weren't visiting her grandmother, we were visiting her entire extended family, they all lived together, cooked, cleaned, worked their farm out back, it was pure magic.

I began to feel like we had walked onto a TV set because there was no *way* that this experience could be real. There were gorgeous abundant fruit trees growing everywhere with the most luscious looking fruits. There was a full farm out back full of fat pigs, chickens, citrus, and everything else you could possibly think of, glory!

Growing there were some fruit's that I recognized like mangos, coconuts and jack fruits, but there were also many fruits that I could not recognize, they were so unique. The type of fruit that you knew only grew in Vietnam and wouldn't be showing up in our local market back in NY anytime soon. Dang… Guess you'll just have to go visit.

It was amazing to take in the whole setting, I couldn't believe my eyes. There was a true magic in that moment arriving to a warm welcome from Kelly's family. We were literally in the middle of nowhere but it didn't feel that way. We had made it to the Mekong Delta baby! And we were experiencing it the way locals did, this was no tourist situation.

As we were wondering around the magical property with Kelly, a boat on the Mekong Delta slowly passed us by with a load of tourists sitting on it looking in. We over heard the tour guide's loud speaker saying that the local life is very simple, that locals live almost completely off the river, and that the area they were passing was very untapped. Just at that moment we began to wave to the boat, realizing how ironic and funny it was that we, two Americans, were standing on the local side, completely out of place and how confused the guide must have been.

When we got settled in we met her family and though they didn't speak any English, they were beyond accommodating and welcoming. It kind of felt like we were celebrities and family all at the same time. I'd never experienced that kind of welcome in my entire life, it was heartwarming.

For as much bliss as the experience was unfortunately the weather on the Mekong was a lot hotter than the city, it was scorching and humid. I was doing my best to stay hydrated but I felt like I was losing the battle. Kelly's cousins, aunts and uncles wanted to take us on a short walk to their farm to show us what they grew as they'd heard that we were chefs from NYC, it was all so sweet, but I was certainly pushing hard to stay with it. The heat normally wouldn't bother me so much but with everything going on with my hormones, I was all out of whack.

When we made the short trek out to their farm I realized it was well worth it. Huge lime trees with fresh limes on them, abundant sugar cane everywhere we looked, I was just in heaven! One of her cousins brought a huge ass knife, a machete of sorts, and chopped some sugar cane down. She split off a couple huge jackfruits, collected a bunch of banana leaves and some other little things that we hadn't seen before and we headed back. Her cousin was a tank, this woman must have been no more than 5 feet tall but she hacked away at the sugar cane like it was no big deal, carrying more than the two of us could carry together.

At this point I should note, our suspicion about how people in Vietnam perceived culture became a reality. When Kelly said that we would be walking to their farm, we were told that it was about 10-15 minutes away by foot but when we made the journey it was more like 3-5 minutes, it was basically their backyard. I have a theory that one of the reasons that people in Vietnam love motorbikes so much is because they seem to think things are a lot further away than we do.

When we got back to the house, Kelly's cousin cut up the sugar cane with her big knife and as we sucked on the sweet treat I tasted heaven in my mouth. It reminded me of being in the sugar cane fields of Ecuador where we all chewed and sucked on the freshest sugar cane, it tasted like the best candy ever. Take that, Starbursts! If you ever have a chance to suck on some fresh sugar cane, I urge you to do so. Once the thick layer of skin is cut by a very sharp knife, the pieces are chopped up into little sticks and then you chew on it releasing the sweet and flavorful juice into your mouth, discarding the pulp once the juice has been released.

Kelly told us that she requested her Grandmother make one of her favorite desserts, it was gluten free and vegan and she said that she thought we would really enjoy it. Her cousin, aunt and great aunt set out to get the necessary ingredients including fresh banana leaves, some rice flours and other ingredients that we didn't recognize. I had no idea what it was going to be but we were excited nonetheless!

While they were gathering goodies for the dessert, the family had a feast waiting for us like I'd never seen before! I tried to get the women to sit down and eat with us but it seemed very clear that only the men, and guests would be sitting at the table to eat while the women continued to cook and clean for the rest of the day.

Kelly told them that I could not eat the food though they tried a few times to get me to eat, but Josh was hungry and had no problem scarfing the meal down. I simply sat down and enjoyed a fresh tea that they had brewed.

On the table, they placed several bowls filled with all sorts of delectable looking dishes. A large plate of unidentified chicken parts with some herbs, a big bowl of fresh herbs, rice porridge with herbs, and freshly cooked rice. The pork was fresh from a pig that they had raised and oddly enough, they did something that would have seemed taboo in America. After they broke down the pork they took some pork shoulder and let it sit out in the sun uncovered, exposed to the world for many hours, they said it helped with the flavor of the meat.

Josh seemed happy eating a feast of food that was as authentic and local as it got. In Ho Chi Minh, even if to us everything seemed quite authentic, this was just straight up a typical meal that they would eat, completely new and exotic in our eyes but perfectly normal and every day in theirs. I watched on as Josh slowly ate away at the feast before him and laughed when they tried to give him more but he said that he was full, they really wanted to feed him until he exploded it seemed. Were they trying to fatten him up for something? No, they just wanted him to eat.

It's funny how much you can talk and communicate just through body language and laughter, food really is the ultimate connector and in this magical moment Josh and I felt all the love. Josh was blown away by the flavors and described everything to me so I did not feel left out.

Afterwards we went to the big market on motorbikes with Kelly and her cousins, she said it was an amazing market that we would love so we were quite excited about that. We jumped on the back of motorbikes that her cousins were riding. They were quite young, maybe 14 years old but somehow, we felt safe. We drove through backroads, riding along the river, laughing and screaming with joy. Riding through the rice paddies on one side and the Mekong and small houses and huts on the other, it felt like we were in a national geographic segment. When we got to the market at first there wasn't much to see, everything was covered by tents and tarps. But when we actually went in we found that the market was huge and filled with food and treats for ages.

One of the first things I noticed was what looked to be large amounts of meat but there was something not quite meaty about it. Kelly explained to us that vegan food was quite popular there because most Buddhists, on certain days of each month, would eat vegetarian and so they have very impressive meat substitutes.

Honestly the bacon looked like bacon, and I don't just mean what we have come to expect in the states as meat substitutes, this was on a whole new level of awesomeness. We bought a nice thick slab of "facon" for me though it was a little weird because it looked and smelled like bacon, even though she assured me it was safe, but I thought it might be fun to maybe try out later that night when we cooked dinner.

As we kept walking we saw a beautiful array of produce and fresh fruits, we bought what we could and kept walking until we found these big logs wrapped in banana leaves. It turns out that they have a variety of fillings, some sweet, some savory, one with banana and steamed rice that was amazing. Oh man, so much great stuff, they were safe for me and delicious. They had a sticky rice filling with different fillings of sweet red beans and other goodies, some savory some sweet. Be sure to check first if you see a treat like this but the good news is there is a chance you can eat it.

★Tip for Eating in Vietnam to Avoid Cross Contamination

As mentioned before if the cart doesn't serve any gluten you can feel safer knowing that there is no cross contamination as most everything is made fresh that day, and they don't use non-stick pans often so the pans can be easily cleaned out but if you want to be extra careful, you might be able to get away with asking someone to cook something for you in a pot that you provided. I know it may seem absurd but there were a few places that we went, especially while hanging with locals, who were more than happy to use our own provided pans.

We kept moving along and saw that they didn't just sell food but all kinds of other little knick-knacks. Already not feeling very well, I ended up buying a mask to go over my mouth as it is very popular way to keep pollution and germs away in Vietnam, so I figured why not? Besides, it was so dusty on motorbikes that I thought it would be fun to try out.

We grabbed a bunch of produce to take to the homestay that we would be staying at next and on our way out of the market I ended up grabbed some treats and cookies to bring back to the children in her family. We were having issues giving gifts to her family members as they seem far more interested in giving than receiving, but considering I am the same way, I was trying to find ways of sneaking in treats and little gifts to show our appreciation for their kindness of taking us in and really making us feel like family, it was a beautiful time.

When we returned to the house we unloaded our groceries and I noticed that Kelly's aunt was sitting on the floor with a big bowl of a blueish looking dough and she was making the special treat that Kelly was raving about. Basically, it is a mix of water, coconut milk and some rice flour that they add the essence of a special leaf that they say smells like a fart. All of a sudden my excitement for the dish went down just a little bit, I had enough unwanted farts between Josh and I to smell, and I felt uneasy about a dessert associated with them. But I figured it had to be good and anyhow, who knows what a Vietnamese fart smells like.

Once the doughy batter is made, they take banana leaves, add a thin layer of the batter in the middle about 6 inches long, wrap it up, steam it, and then they serve it with fresh thickened coconut milk.

It was an experience like none other I'd ever had and I even got to make and steam the treats with them. It was a true family effort, only the woman made it as the men hung out and spoke to one another. Both young and old, all the woman and kids sat around, laughing and making treats. Josh serenaded us all by playing the ukulele which they seemed to really enjoy. When it came time to eat I was blown away, it was so delicious, tasted nothing like a fart, and how could something be called a fart leaf? It had been hot by the river and I was struggling to keep it together but the moment I tasted the treat I suddenly felt like myself again.

One of the most exciting parts of this experience was that there was no gluten to be found in their entire household. They ate a lot of rice, meat, vegetables, fruits, fish, but they simply didn't not cook with gluten which made me automatically feel much safer and that really added to the whole dining experience.

I will note that it was extremely hot and seeing as how my body had already been taking a beating with everything going on I was starting to feel a little better. Perhaps still a bit dehydrated, but maybe it was just a matter of getting used to the heat. After all, we came from what was one of the worst winters I had ever experienced in New York and we were thrown into the middle of summer in Vietnam, so my body was all over the place.

After we were done snacking on this delicious food, I wasn't feeling up to cooking for myself, and besides I was so full from the treat. So, we were taken over to the pagoda next door where we met two monks. These monks were making something very special, cooking in large pots, putting the pots in the water to cool the liquid down. It turns out they were making actual grass jelly, a process that involves taking the special grass, washing it, cooking it in water, straining it with added water, and then cooking it again until it jelled up.

The monks are very poor we learnt through Kelly and it is through donations and selling this grass jelly that they make enough money to survive. They dedicate themselves to their practice in serving their community. It is a long, slow and arduous process of making the jelly but they did it with a smile on their face and seemed quite peaceful.

We wanted to give back in some way and so we gave $100 to the monks as a sealed donation, they didn't know that at the time but we felt it was a good thing to do and we knew that it would go a long way for them. It felt like the right thing to do as Kelly told us that one of their monks had fallen ill so they were working extra hard to make more grass jelly in order to take care of him. They wanted to give us some of their grass jelly so we got a big bag full of it to take with us on our next journey. They also told us that this grass jelly had a cooling effect on the body for the hot weather.

Though I was certainly not feeling 100%, almost like I was in some heat driven dream, just sitting around watching the boats go by the river and getting to connect with Kelly and her family was wonderful. Being able to cook with them, watching how they cooked and seeing the beautiful food that they crafted and the family dynamic of it all, was truly surreal. Here I had not expected much and yet ended up with a down to earth and authentic experience that was such a blessing to be a part of. Just having the chance to see how they lived life out there was wonderful. It peaceful in a way but it seemed to be a lot of hard work, everything was made and built from scratch. They even used the little river next to their house as garbage (although that seemed a little weird), they just tossed everything right in it!

Before we left they fed us one more meal, a beautiful dish with slow cooked pork that they had cooked all day. This was the pork that they leave out in the sun for a full day to tenderize before they cook it. There were hard boiled eggs that they cook in the pork broth and a variety of noodles and other little plates.

I, of course was not able to eat because I was still stuffed from the fart leaf dessert but I was happy to sit down and share in the experience. I brought out some vegetables to munch on and enjoyed watching the others eat a wonderfully prepared meal. The woman did not eat with the men, the men sat down, plus Kelly and I, as we were guests, and the woman seemed to keep bringing out more and more food. They kept trying to get us to eat more, saying that we did not eat enough and that we needed to eat more. The women kept filling up Josh's bowl, it was never ending, it was amazing! But at some point, we really had to just cut it off because they would probably feed Josh until he passed out from a food coma!

There were two fruits that were completely worth mentioning, things that if happen to come across, you absolutely must try! One was like a Pomelo or a large grapefruit, the skin was peeled off, each juicy wedge separated and it was served with a mixture of chili and a little sugar. Instead of taking bites of it you rip out pieces of flesh and sprinkle on the chili mixture if you'd like. It was so fresh and satisfying. There was a fruit that didn't have a translation really but Kelly called it 'The Bell Fruit' as it was red and looked kind of like a bell. It tasted like a mix between an apple and a juicy plum, it was to die for and seeing as how they grew all over the property we gathered as many as we could for later.

Right before we left to head to our homestay we were taken to Kelly's Aunt's house down the street to pick up some fruits that Kelly would be taking back with her family. It was quite a vision to see her house, she had some beautiful fruit trees and they had us taste these small round fruits that reminded us of lychee without the spikes, similar texture inside but the fruit was sour and delicious.

We cut down fresh coconuts and got to sip on their refreshingly intoxicating water inside, and her aunt hacked off the biggest jack fruit I had ever seen on a tree for Kelly to take back to her mom. It was jackfruit season and you could smell its pungent aroma whenever you were near a tree.

When we went back to her house we took a picture with the entire family, they were all so adorable and sweet. We said our goodbyes and then Kelly and her dad took us to the bus station. That was when things got weird.

Chapter 10:

Freaked Out at the Bus Station

We heard from some friends who had traveled to Vietnam that there were two forms of basic bus transportation, one for the locals, and one for tourists. The prices are basically the same, and the routes are similar, but we were told to always take the tourist bus. We weren't sure why but from what we had heard the local bus wasn't a good way to get a more authentic experience or meet locals and it was best to take the tourist bus.

When Kelly's dad took us to the bus station he told us to wait inside while he squared away the bus details, this was sweet since the car ride had been long and I needed to tinkle it up. The bathroom even had toilet paper. Sweet! Talk about my favorite luxury... It was really kind of him to make our travel arrangements, but also a little anxiety driven - what would happen once he left? It appeared that no one spoke English at the bus terminal, we were the only foreigners it seemed for miles, how would we carry on after they left? Would we get taken advantage of? Or would we magically be taken care of by the universe like we always were? These were the funny thoughts running through my mind... All these racing thoughts as I reached into my bag for my wallet.

I paid for the two bus tickets and then he said that we should wait, that once the bus arrived, one of the workers would let us know and point us to the bus. This seemed easy enough, but it being late at night and in a desolate location so I couldn't help but have a little fear creep in. Besides we were beat down from a magical day, it was hot and there are people everywhere with little kids screaming... I prayed and asked that all would be well, praying never hurt anything after all. I didn't want us to get kidnapped, robbed and thrown into a river in a bag or something —what can I say? Growing up my sister would trick me into watching horror films...

Absurd and illogical thoughts aside, when Kelly and her father told us we were all set we thanked them for what seemed like about a million times for the incredible journey, said our goodbyes, and took a seat in the bus station on the bright green slippery plastic chairs.

The first thing that I noticed while we were sitting there, was that this was a nice bus station. There were food vendors and shops all around with some enticing looking food to buy. The second thing that I noticed was that the station was made up of pretty much all locals, and then it dawned on me—seeing as how we were at a random bus station and not in a major city, it was very likely that this was a local bus station with no tourists' buses. Not that that was a big deal, but it was our first time really off the beaten path, alone, no phones, surrounded by no one that speaks the language, with all our expensive camera gear, just waiting... Trusting that it would all work out, though admittedly a little nervous.

After about 15 minutes of waiting Josh went to the counter to ask about the bus, they looked at our ticket as though they didn't know why we were there, even though they had just seen us with Kelly's dad just minutes before, they handed us two bottled waters and told us to wait. We waited another 15 minutes and she waved at us letting us know that our bus was coming soon.

We went outside with all our bags which at this point in the night felt like carrying a million things while trying to balance it all on one of those circus tricycles that are far too small for any adult. As we waited for the right bus to arrive, I hoped that I would know which one it was and not end up on the wrong bus to who knows where. When the next bus pulled up we saw the driver get out and begin to let people on. We got in line, showed our ticket to the driver and he told us to put our luggage under the bus, score! We were finally on our way—the universe had heard my prayer and was like girl, I got you! We put our luggage under the bus and got back in line to get on the bus, excited that all we had to do now was sit.

However, when we got to the front of the line the driver told us to stand on the side and to not get on. I was confused as to why and I asked what was going on.

"You wait here, no get on the bus," He said, looking a little annoyed as though my very presence was annoying to him.

"What do you mean we don't get on the bus? I said. "We bought a ticket, our stuff is under the bus," I was waving the ticket and pointing to our luggage under the bus, starting to get a little nervous. This went on for a few minutes when all of a sudden a local Vietnamese man around 25 years old who spoke good English came up to us.

"Please," he said. "You must wait here while the other people get on the bus."

"But why?" I said. "I bought a ticket, our luggage is under the bus."

"Please, just wait here while the other people get on, that is just the way that it is here."

Confused, tired, hot and now irritated, I looked to Josh and he told me just to wait and that it would be fine. We waited until everyone got on the bus and finally, to our confused relief, the bus driver let us get on the bus. I must confess that the experience was odd and unsettling, it made me feel like I was being treated unfairly and put down for being an outsider, like I had been as a child.

Growing up half Ecuadorean I always felt judged by some of the kids I went to school with. Nothing more than ignorant comments from children repeating things, most likely from their parents, about how I was a "wet-bag," and that I should be mowing their lawns and fixing up their house. Looking back, I know it was just their own insecurities and upbringing but at the time it stung.

Kelly's dad had mentioned for us to tell the bus driver our destination and that the driver would drive us directly there. We made sure to do that on the way onto the bus, he slightly smiled, nodded his head, as though to say that he got it, and that all was okay.

We found a seat somewhere in the middle of the bus and began to settle down into our seats but just as we sat down we were told that we must move our stuff and sit in the back of the bus. Feeling even more irritated and helpless, we quietly got up and moved to the back. In the back, there was a set of 3 open seats that we quietly took and settled in.

At this point I wasn't feeling very good about the whole bus situation. Our bags were under the bus, we were the only tourists on the bus, hardly anyone spoke English and it didn't feel like there wasn't much interest for anyone to want to be of help to us —this was a big shift from the warm welcome and stay we had with Kelly's family. It was all very strange and made me uncomfortable, however this was not the first time I have traveled outside the U.S and I've been in dangerous and shady situations so I did my best to sit back, relax, get through the bus ride and remember that I was an outsider and sometimes that means being treated differently.

We sat ever so quietly on the hour or so bus ride, tired, a little uncomfortable, but being sure to stay awake. Most of the people on the bus fell fast asleep, the others minded their own business. It became clear that any danger or prejudice I felt was not going to be an actual threat. It was late, everyone probably wanted to simply get to where they were going.

After about an hour, the bus driver's assistant started going back and asking people something which we later realized was their location drop off. Slowly, as we reached the final bus destination in Can Thon, one by one, the bus would stop and start to let people off. After about 5 stops the bus pulled into a large bus terminal, the lights came on, and everyone got off.

Confused and not knowing if they had passed our stop, on top of not knowing where in the heck we were, we got off the bus, grabbed our things and asked the local who helped us out before what was going on. He said that the bus offers free transportation to your destination as long as it is within 10 miles of the station.

We went inside, address in hand, hoping we were not far off from our destination, and went up to the reception. The lady looked at the address for a while, it was hard to tell if she knew where it was or not and we semi-patiently waited to get a clear answer. The bus station was open to the hot muggy thick almost like butter air, it was overcrowded and as the multiple t.v.'s blasted with noise all from different channels it felt a bit like hell...

The Vietnamese woman working at the station stared at our paper, for what felt like forever, where the address was scribbled, squinting and looking confused as though it wasn't really an address. My discomfort and frustration started to boil again. I tried to remind myself that everything always works out, that we were fine, that we were being tested for our patience but clearly, I needed to work on this because Josh was cool as a cucumber...

So many teachings for me on this night of travel—to have more compassion and patience for situations out of my control, to remember that it always works out. Funny enough, one of the biggest reasons I fell in love with traveling to foreign countries in the first place was to grow in that area.

After about ten minutes of confusion we gave her the telephone number to the homestay where we were to spend the next couple nights and she called them up. They spoke for a while and while we waited an English-speaking local came over to try and help. It turned out he was a doctor and had done a residency in the US. His name was An, which means peace, and coincidentally him helping us translate sure did bring us a lot of peace. When the receptionist got off the phone and spoke with An he told us that our homestay was a very weird location, that they didn't know where it was, and that we should get a cab from the station. He claimed that the cab drivers would know where it was and to make sure to get a green cab. Not knowing what else to do and since it was really late at night, we decided to have faith and trust that he was guiding us in the right direction.

Feeling as lost as ever, but also hopeful because a total stranger had shown us such kindness, we grabbed our stuff and went outside to get a cab. Within seconds a slew of cab drivers came up to us all at the time saying, "Where are you going? I will take you anywhere, very good price, yes."

I was overwhelmed but it was also quite comical, we were fish out of water, past the point of exhaustion. We noticed none of the drivers who approached us were in green cabs, the ones that are said to be safest in Vietnam, so we said no thank you and kindly waved them away. But as we walked away one of the drivers came up to us, he seemed very adamant.

"See, see, meter, yes, taxi, same same, all same," he said.

From the looks of it his car did look legit, which is important in Vietnam as lots of people with regular cars will try to rip you off. Josh showed him the location and we gave him the homestay phone number. The cab driver called and talked to them for a bit and then said he knew where to go. Josh and I looked at each other, I tilted my head a little bit, unsure of what to think, he nodded at me, I nodded back, and we got in the car. In minutes, we were off, driving into the unknown, again having that trust and faith in our hearts that everything was going to be fine even if our heads were a little unsure.

There is something about driving late at night that is always a bit uncomfortable in a foreign place, it's dark, every turn you make you are watching to see if where the driver is going looks like a busy and safe road, your senses are majorly heightened.

Growing up in Ecuador, I always heard the stories of tourists who were taken to a strange place, robbed, or worse, tortured and killed. A bit extreme I know, my parents were foreigners and didn't trust many people, but even if those stories were rare and used mostly just to scare me to make me aware of where I was and what could happen if I wasn't vigilant about my surroundings, I have become a hyper aware person. Even though my heart was racing a little, unsure of where we would end up on this night, as I squeezed Josh's hand tightly, I knew that nothing was going to happen to us.

As we drove on, we went from seeing a busy Can Thon city, to slowly entering into a more and more rural area, passing fields, driving down dirt roads in the nearly pitch dark. Our driver was driving pretty slowly and he seemed relaxed and confident like he knew where he was going. With almost no sign of civilization in sight I began to pray for protection. "We'll be there soon," whispered Josh into my ear in a calming and loving tone, "then we can shower and rest sweetheart." This brought me some peace that only the one who you truly can bring.

We drove further and further down the small dirt road until we finally pulled up to a wooden sign sticking out of the ground. The driver parked the car and signaled that this was the place even though it looked like we were in a random empty field. In good faith, we paid him a little reluctantly because there were no bright lights, nothing really that signified we had arrived, but we got out, grabbed our things, and began walking over a narrow bamboo bridge which seemed to be the entrance to our homestay.

We read that the place we were staying had incredibly good reviews but so far, we saw nothing but trees and plants. As we slowly walked over the bridge and down the winding paved road we crossed through a field and were in what felt like a mini jungle. It was gorgeous, and a bit scary in what felt like, but I kept my head up high even though it felt like my heart was pounding right out of my chest.

As we got closer we heard more and more voices until finally we found the entrance to the homestay. Wow, for as shady and sketchy as our car ride and trip had been, all the fear, anxiety and discomfort dissolved the moment we arrived at our beautiful homestay nestled right in the heart of a tiny jungle of lush greenery. For the next two days, we would be staying at a serene and secluded small homestay comprised of little more than six small huts for visitors made from little more than bamboo, thatch and local organic materials.

It was a green homestay meaning that they used recyclable goods, kept a local water source, and everything they served and provided us with was local which was nice. When we walked in we noticed a big open dining space that had four or so dining tables where some guests were hanging out, laughing and merrily chatting away. There was a small kitchen where some food was being prepared, and a reception desk where a sweet and petite woman named Linh patiently waited for our arrival. Right next to her there was a large glass jar with snakes in some sort of liquid just chilling on the table like it was totally normal which immediately made me think of the Anthony Bourdain episode in Vietnam I once saw where he drank snake blood and liquor for male potency or something like that.

The peaceful and serene homestay held no more than 20 people, it was truly a small tropical paradise covered by wild fruits of all types—pineapples were growing out front, coconut trees stood tall lining the outside borders of the place, each giving of a naturally sweet aroma in the air, bringing a magical sense of romance. To top it all off, we were dead smack in the middle of a huge rice paddy under a bright blanket of cosmic stars staring down at us with their infinite wisdom.

Linh, our homestay host, greeted us and asked if we were hungry in a quiet and broken English. We thanked her but said we had a long day and simply wanted to shower and rest. As she showed us to our rustic hut she told us to make ourselves at home and to just ask her if we needed anything at all. We thanked her kindly, tossed our luggage in the room and I plopped right on the bed.

Josh, wanted to make the most of our few days down south, spoke to the host about taking a boat trip the next day. One of our biggest intentions and hope for traveling to the Mekong Delta was influenced by a video we had seen from a famous Vietnamese Chef. In the video the host took out a sampan, or small river boat, and traveled through the famous floating market where locals sell all sorts of fresh fruits, meats, and vegetables, and cooked while he glided down the river. How cool would it be if we could attempt a similar feat and cook a delectably fresh meal of vegan and gluten free yummies, I wondered.

The very idea of floating in a small boat, collecting and preparing fresh food with our little burner just sounded too good to pass up. We had heard there were a few different floating markets on the Mekong Delta. Cai Rang was the bigger and more popular one where boats filled with tourists went to watch the market come alive at the crack of dawn. Cai Rang, though a sight to see, wasn't a place to go and attempt to buy food to cook. The food they sold was mostly to locals, wholesale, bulk produce and the like, tourists only went to watch the action unfold, awesome, but not for us.

After some googling we had found out that there was another floating market called Phong Dien that is located not too far, somewhere south-west, of Can Tho. It is slightly smaller than Cai Rang, but worth a visit—especially since it is less popular for tourists, a total score for those, like us, who are seeking a more authentic experience. We were informed that with a little luck you could hire a small boat and go up to some people in the market and buy a wide range of fresh produce. Yes, this is where we wanted to go, the idea of being able to get off the beaten path and see ingredients that maybe we hadn't before, to see the perhaps foods that were native to this part of the country and never made it to the states, for us both, as chefs and food lovers, goodness was this idea exciting!

Aside from some information online we didn't have any leads before getting to our homestay meaning we had no solid arrangement and plan to go to the floating market the next morning. Luckily, as Josh found out, the homestay took their own private boat to the floating market. The only problem was they left at six a.m. the next morning and didn't get back until noon and it was our only chance to go before we left the homestay since we had an early flight the following day. We were super exhausted from traveling, I was stressed from the night before, it was late and the heat was no less extreme in the middle of the jungle. I wasn't sure if I would be able to peel my sorry butt out of bed that early but I did my best to take a quick shower before jumping back into bed and attempting to get some rest.

I should add that at this point I was feeling terrible from the heat, hormone imbalance and travel, it was making me extremely emotional. That night when we got in tried my best to hold back what I felt boiling inside but I simply couldn't anymore, everything felt like a water line waiting to burst and I intuitively knew the only way out was to break down and release the excess energy and emotion pent up. This was challenging on my ego because we were only literally a few feet away from the other people staying there, separated by a thin bamboo wall, where I could hear their every word, listening to them chatting away and having a lively time, laughing loud like hyenas, their giggles cutting through the emotions swelling in my throat, causing my hands to tremble with emotion like an old washing machine jerking this way and that...

Feeling trapped as if there was no place for me to go for privacy, I grabbed several pillows and shoved my face deep into the fluffy clouds, trying to suffocate the waling that was pouring out of my mouth. I made every attempt to mute the horrid sounds expelling out of my mouth, like a killer trying to suffocate his victim, I realized that they would probably hear my anyhow. The little voice inside my head seemed to be playing tricks on me. It was like a tiny mouse in a suit pointing at me, screaming and doing itS best to convince me that the other guests would think I was a lunatic for crying and screaming the moment I showed up in paradise. For some reason in that moment I really didn't want to give the wrong impression, they didn't know what was wrong with me, what would they really think? Looking back, I am not sure why I even cared but I suppose when one reaches the point of emotional and physical exhaustion all reason fly's out the door.

I continued to swell with emotion like a tidal wave, crashing again and again on the shore of hopeless hell... The more I released the tears inside, the more I bullied myself for not being in control of myself. I felt terrible and out of control with no hope in sight— my legs like sausages that had burst in a boiling pot of oil, my body so swollen that when I looked down I saw what appeared to be the feet of an elephant, I just couldn't take it, it was too much. I sat on the floor in front of the bed while Josh showered, holding the pillow tight against my face desperately trying to silence my wailing and sobbing.

In that moment, everything happening to me all at once, I couldn't help but think of my dad. I missed him immensely and the more I thought about him the more I shook to the core with grief. Josh came out of the shower stunned to find me on the floor, seeing me trying to muffle my cries. He dropped to his knees beside me and took me in his arms, holding me, telling me it was alright. I wanted to feel comforted by him but I felt so uncomfortable and irritable that I didn't know what to do. I was so swollen and bloated that I couldn't recognize my feet or ankles anymore, couldn't see the separation between my toes, it was awful, almost as if my once skinny toes were now stuffed together like grape leaves. Was I in my own personal hell? Josh seemed totally fine and good with the heat and traveling but here I was, blabbering like a baby on the floor in what should have been a very beautiful place, missing my dad and feeling like I had elephantiasis...

When the rainworms stopped, we attempted to get to sleep, but hearing the loud conversations of the other people outside my small wooden window was making me more and more irritated, I just wanted peace and quiet. I took another cold shower which seemed to sooth my emotions and help with the swelling. I took some time to breath in the shower and think about what was really going on. Talking about the day with Josh and remembering that this moment was temporary it started to bring me great solace, seeing that what was going on in my head and heart was just a teaching to prepare me for what was ahead in life.

I was starting to calm down when I got back in bed and hoped to get some decent rest. The next adventure of the night was trying to keep the mosquito tent around us tucked in tight to keep the bugs out. The net was far too small for the bed so I put socks on because I knew how much mosquitos loved my ankles and feet, take that you little blood suckers! The bed was made from some sort of recycled wood and other local materials, on the website it looked plush and quite luxurious but in person it didn't feel like there was any padding or that it was a bed at all. It may not have bothered me on any normal day but this was no normal day, to say the least.

We may have been in paradise from the looks of it, but bugs buzzing in your ears while you try to rest, sweat beading down on your face like pearls fresh from the ocean as you toss in bed trying to keep distance from your hot and sticky partner who you wish you could be cuddling with, surely felt otherwise. Some romantic time would have been nice but at this point I would settle for a moment of peace and quiet as I attempted to rest my head.

"I love you beso," I said. "I'm sorry I'm in such a state but I know tomorrow will be a better day. Let's just let this moment end and set the intention for tomorrow to be epic."

In my mind, I couldn't help but wonder where the end adventure button, or the stop rider here lever, was located, what did I need to do to step off this journey? I wanted out but with no cell phone, no sense of direction, no car, no nothing, I was stuck and besides I didn't want to be without my lover. In that moment, I realized the end button was to think of how grateful I was to have Josh in my life and how something as simple as that was worth more than I could have dreamed of.

Accommodation Tips

When traveling, you have any number of places you can stay. and rent on a fair budget. From hostels where you are likely to meet other travels and rent on the cheap, to hotels that are often pricier but offer you an easy way to check in, book tours and taxis, information desk, breakfast and cleaning service, to sites like AirBnB where you can rent a home or apartment and live a bit more like a local.

The homestay option ended up being great for us on the trip, it was a lovely way, in the end, to get to experience a more authentic stay, meet *fellow travelers, as well as interact with locals who could show you what life was really like, especially in more rural and untapped areas. The benefit of staying with someone who speaks the local tongue and has lived there for many years really opens up new doors. If you have a fairly long trip I suggest you consider a few different options, switch up your accommodations from place to place, see what works best for you.*

Chapter 11:

Heaven and Hello!

When I finally managed to wake up the next day I was glad to hear the silence. Josh was not in the room but he came back quickly, walking in and telling me that he was just served breakfast. Breakfast was of course the three things that I used to love most, the three things that I could not even think about eating again unless I wanted to be near death and on a very "special" roller coaster whose seat looked a lot like a toilet. A baguette, a fried egg and cheese was the standard breakfast menu served each and every morning as we came to find out. They served a nice warm baguette with a fried egg and some baby bell cow soft cheese in a little tin foil thing. I used to eat the shit out of that meal when I was young, a whole baguette to myself with a liter of ice cold whole milk and a twelve, yes twelve egg omelet — Josh seems to think that my food allergies came from eating way too much of the things I loved most as a child.

When I finally peeled myself out of bed to take a shower and get some stretching in I started to feel slightly better, the tears were gone, and I kept reminding myself that everything was going to be okay. After a slow start and a fresh breakfast of fruit from the homestay which they graciously prepared for me when I told them I could not eat the standard breakfast, we decided to take a bike ride seeing as how we missed the early boat to the floating market. I wasn't sure what my energy levels would be like in the heat but I thought getting a little physical activity would do me well, getting some much-needed feel good endorphins into my body to boost my mood and to help with releasing water weight seemed like a great idea at the time. I had a window of decent health and I wanted to seize the moment!

We grabbed some bamboo hats from the front desk, jumped on the bikes and were off down a small path that lead to the main road. As we started to ride away one of the workers from our homestay spotted us and waved us to follow him. He was a cheerful Vietnamese man that hardly spoke any English. The night before Josh and I overheard one of the other guests refer to him as Mr. Hello as it seemed that the only word he knew in English was "hello." He would use the word "hello" with a myriad of different hand gestures, facial expressions and inflections of his voice to express different things. "Hello" could mean literally anything for him. With a hand wave, it could mean a simple hello, with a hand shake it could be a halting stop or to be careful, or it could even be a "hello" with his hands mimicking the process of eating food to see if you were hungry.

In this instance, it seemed like he wanted to point us in the direction of town as he yelled from his motorbike "hello, hello," while waving us to follow him down the road. As we road down the dusty street, the same street that seemed so silent, almost creepy the same road from the night before, it started to show its signs of life in the daylight. What was once very unassuming and seemed mostly of farm land quickly became little shops, restaurants, fruit stands and bars. As we peddled on, my energy starting to bubble back and I felt optimistic about my first real physical activity in days. Riding down the road I noticed a small garlic factory with about ten women peeling garlic. I got a wife of its pungent smell in my face. Garlic is of course great for warding off vampires but it's all great to eat as it helps fight off sickness and infections.

Further down the road we saw fresh sugar cane juice being pressed, farmers were working in the fields, picking vegetables and rice. It was so picturesque like a scene out of a movie. Suddenly I felt a wave of positivity, my strength was coming back and I started to feel great!

We continued to follow Mr. Hello on his motorbike as he sped on by and eventually led us out of the path and onto a main road near a gas station and the freeway. We made a sharp right turn and before we knew it we were peddling on a narrow road between the river and local houses surrounded by green. We passed through tree after tree seeing fresh jackfruit, coconut and mango trees everywhere, the air was intoxicating with the aroma of sweet fruits. I was in my fruit fantasy, we could have just ripped fruits down and eaten like sweet savages but we kept on peddling unsure of who owned the fruits. Every so often as Mr. Hello's bike went out of sight he would stop and circle back to make sure we were okay and close in sight.

After about thirty minutes of peddling down by the river my chain got caught and fell off my bike. As we pulled over and started to figure out how to fix it, a local boy came up to us, grabbed a stick, and without saying anything, with a simple smile and a few gestures of his hands he put the chain back on the bike in no time and we were back on our way. The pure generosity of just wanting to help almost brought me to tears, you don't really see that kind of kindness in the states anymore.

When we finally made a right turn, and popped back on the original road, we decided to stay out, we were both feeling good and we were not ready to turn back. We biked for a while and ended up stopping at what seemed to be a local bar of sorts. The lady there had a standard sugar cane juice press and so we ordered two cold ones. This is nothing like having sugar cane growing up in Ecuador – where were would visit sugar cane factories in the jungle and be given big sticks of sugar cane to chew on like we had with Kelly's family. Here they fed the whole sugar cane through a round metal press that crushes it, extracting the sweet yellowish green juices. As the sugar cane goes through the press they fold it over itself and run it through again and again until all the juice is extracted. It's hard to describe what the drink tastes like, it is very sweet that is for sure, and there is almost a nutty flavor too it, but it is so refreshing and rejuvenating

After we finished our second round of sugar cane juice (we just couldn't get enough) we jumped on our bikes and headed back. Along the way, we saw a fresh produce stand and new this was our chance to grab some food so we could cook later. The following day we would be taking an early flight all the way to the capital city Hanoi and I wanted to be prepared in case there was no food for me to eat.

We had some nice treats from the day before from Kelly's place with vegetables that we had bought at the market but we couldn't resist buying some fresh fruit and herbs from the adorable little lady standing on the side of the road, she must have been in her late 80's if not older but in great shape so of course, seeing as how it costs about nothing for all of the food she was selling, it was a no brainer to stock up on goodies.

When we got back I was feeling probably the best I had felt on the entire trip and I was ready to do an epic cooking jam as well as some overdue face stuffing with yummy food. The morning boat trip had not come back yet with all the other hotel guests so I was happy to bask in quiet stillness. I started chopping up food and sautéing some vegetables on a chair with our flexible cutting board on our front porch. No need to make anything too fancy, I just wanted to get some fresh food in our bellies that we both could enjoy. We were cooking outdoors which as a couple is one of our favorite things to do together, everything was as local as could be and I knew it would all taste delicious together as we were cooking with love and gratitude. We had an array of fresh vegetables and spices that we had bought earlier that day as well as collected the days before. Some of it, like the carrots and beets, was recognizable, while other things, like this odd green leafy plant, I had never seen before and was excited to see how it tasted.

★Tip for Cooking Random Ingredients★

What might be completely foreign to you, is a very normal ingredient for someone who lives in the place that it grows. When shopping at the market I always find it a great idea to get a mixture of ingredients that you are familiar with as well as grab a few things you have never cooked, or seen, before. You can try an ask the person selling what the name of it is so you can look it up when you have internet access, but in many cases, they will give you basic instructions as to how to cook it.

We found often that the person selling the food would say things like "very good if you fry," or "eat fresh," simple commands to give us a basic jumping point. A quick web search is always helpful when you know the name of the ingredient but sometimes you will find something that is so exotic that no one has ever written about how to cook it. If you are unsure of what to do, don't hesitate to ask a local for some tips or use your intuition. Typically boiling or stir frying a vegetable you have never seen before with a little salt and maybe some chili is a good start to understanding its purpose in the field of deliciousness.

As I cooked along, stir frying some of the veggies, making a raw salad after peeling some of the others, Josh filming and capturing all the action, some of the other guests started to arrive from their boat trip and were quite curious as to what we were doing. We had asked Linh, woman running the kitchen, if we could use some of her pots for cooking, she said we were welcome to use the kitchen as we liked but we told her we only needed a large pot to make a few things.

Since this was a homestay we made sure to clear it with her first before cooking on the porch, just to be respectful. She was more than willing to let us use her kitchen but the lighting wasn't very good in there so we were happy to hear that she was okay with us cooking outside our room. She wanted to check out what we were doing, she seemed very interested, it was quite cute, she stood and watched as we cooked away asking some questions but mostly staring with a curious look on her face as if she was thinking "Hmm, I've never seen someone cook here, this is quite interesting." It's comical trying to read someone's thoughts from a different culture when language is not there to communicate.

When we finished cooking we ate a beautiful meal sitting outside in the dining area; stir fried greens, a yellow veggie curry of sorts, a raw carrot and beet salad with a tangy lime dressing, it was really shaping up to be a great day. On top of that, after being let down that we had missed our chance to visit, and possibly cook, at the floating market, we received some good news.

It turns out that even though I overslept and missed the first boat ride, our homestay offered a private Sampan boat tour for us to go through the Mekong Delta for only three dollars a person. While we ate, we met a middle aged German couple who were quite friendly who said they would be joining us on the journey.

After lunch, we cleaned up, relaxed, and around 4pm we took a short walk (again they said about 15 minutes and it was more like 5) to the river, jumped on a boat with Mr. Hello at the helm and the five of us were off to see the magical river that was the home to thousands of Vietnamese people.

As we slowly sped along on our Sampan, (which is just a long and narrow boat that seats about five, with a small motor and rudder on the back), we all felt quite at peace. Dragonflies' were overhead, which was powerful because in almost every part of the world dragonflies symbolize change and change in the perspective of self-realization, the kind of change that has its source in mental and emotional maturity and the understanding of the deeper meaning of life. So, I knew deep inside things were about to take a turn for the better not just in our trip but our relationship, and our lives, at that moment I never felt more loved and at peace with myself and my lover. The water was smooth and calm, though it wasn't clear water and you couldn't see any fish or anything, the feeling of floating on the river in a small boat near the ground with the views of everyday life felt very Zen and healing.

We slowly started to see where Mr. Hello got his favorite word from, for anytime a child saw us cruising the river they would scream out in excitement, "HELLO! HELLO!" It put a smile on our faces, such a small genuine gesture can create waves of joy throughout your entire being.

Seeing the children's excitement was moving but what really pulled our interest was what life on the river was really like for locals. People would be cleaning their clothing, washing themselves in the river, taking a dip, and working hard. It was arduous in some ways, peaceful in others, and often repetitive work living on the river but it was nice to see. I suppose it is what you would expect from life on a river but it was a great reminder to us for while our lives are busy and fulfilling, sometimes the peaceful side of connecting to the roots of humanity and nature really holds the key to true happiness and contentment.

When we got back from our trip we cleaned up with a cold shower and sat down for a large family style dinner. We had prepared some extra food for me earlier, I always make more than enough for multiple meals, so I could sit in on the family meal and munch on my own food. It was fun coming to dinner with different food than anyone else because it opens a door to teach others who are interested in what food allergies and Celiac Disease are which is a true blessing once you learn and empower yourself. Everyone was very curious and sweet, their food also looked delicious. A vegetable noodle soup made with cabbage, pineapples, tamarind, whole pieces of fish, fresh rice noodles, fresh herbs, and of course fresh rice paper (which if you put it in your mouth would just melt).

The rice paper that they had was incredible, it was also one of the few things that I felt safe eating because I knew what it was made of, how it was made and knew there was no chance of cross contamination as most places that make rice paper only make rice products. This rice paper was unlike anything I have ever had before, I still dream of it. Unlike in the states where you have dried out rice paper that you must hydrate in water to use, this rice paper was so thin and translucent, it was almost like a clear piece of paper delicate and yet resilient, it didn't just fall apart in your hand but you could easily roll it up and eat it as if it was a little crepe without wetting it first. It reminded me of fresh pasta in a fun way. It was fresh, and it added the perfect texture of chewiness to a meal that without it would not have been as satisfying. I hoped to find it wherever else that we went to keep the food texture game and meal enjoyment high, I had never had anything quite so satisfying!

We finished up dinner, had a nice chat with the German couple from the river boat tour, Sara and Adler, who seemed very passionate and knowledgeable about food and different dishes in Germany, which is always fun to talk about and learn from others while traveling. They even knew a few people in Germany who had gluten intolerance as well so they were intrigued by how effortlessly we seemed to travel together and sharing meals with others, we shared our tips and tricks with them to inspire their friends. After the day, full of activities, we were feeling pooped and went to our room, packed our things and got in bed, we knew we had a long day of travel the next morning so we wanted to be sure that we could get some proper rest.

Packing and Traveling Tips

While we had initially planned to take the train or bus up north, we found that flying was not only cheap but easy. There are two main airports, one in Hanoi and the other in Ho Chi Minh but there was another, large, airport near the homestay that offered an easy flight to Hanoi. Taking a train is a fun and scenic way to get a taste of the city, you can take an overnight train and skip on a hotel for the night, leaving in the late afternoon or early evening and usually arriving the following morning, but it all depends on how you like to travel. Being on a train for 16 hours can be a lot for some people.

A great tip for packing is to try and pack as much as you can the night before you head out, especially if you have an early flight. Leave out clothing that you will need for the following day and have everything tucked away as well as have your flight information printed out or downloaded on your device. You might be tired and want to crash right into bed but getting to sleep in or wake up and get a stretch and work out in, not having to worry about packing and getting ready helps for an anxiety free travel day.

Chapter 12:

Hanoi Brings Joy

The next morning, we woke up early and had some breakfast before our flight. Josh had the homestay staple— baguette with cheese, two fried eggs, some bread and butter, not authentically Vietnamese in anyway but still delicious in his eyes, while I had a simple yet refreshing and vibrant breakfast of dragon fruit mixed with chia and flax that I bloomed in green tea for extra flavor, and a side of protein powder mixed with water, loads of water, to stay hydrated. After breakfast, we showered, finished packing a few of our traveling kitchen utensils and jumped into a cab to catch our flight to Hanoi. We were both buzzing with excitement, the eco homestay was great but we were ready for some a/c and a real comfy bed.

On this occasion we were lucky because a new airport had recently opened close to where we had been staying. Can Tho international airport wasn't as big as the two major city airports but it was all shiny and new and saved us a trip back to Ho Chi Minh city. The airport may have been small but it was nice and clean and it even had air conditioning which in all honestly, I had been missing. To make things even more awesome is that when we arrived there was virtually no line to get through to the gate, yahoo!

Just to give you an idea of how fast it was to get checked in, we arrived at the airport an hour before our flight and managed to check in and go through security in about ten minutes flat. It turned out I couldn't bring my mini scissors (which we used to cut herbs and god knows what else) in my carry-on bag so I decided to check them instead of throwing them out. I had to go out through security, rechecked another bag, go back through security again and we still had about 40 minutes before our flight took off. Talk about airport wizardry!

We noticed that in the airport they were selling some odd things, at least for the airport standards we had come to know, things like big bags of sprawling produce and other colorful foods, objects you would never see in the states. Of course, only in Vietnam could you get your bulk veggie shopping on before catching a flight. They also had interesting candies that I could hardly recognize as well as a bunch of fancy jewelry to buy for a good price. While fancy jewelry wasn't in our budget, we couldn't help ourselves when we saw they had dried jackfruit chips, we snagged a couple bags for the ride, it was lucky for me that they were only jackfruit, one of my favorite funky, tropical and crunchy treats.

The flight was short and sweet, it took around two hours from almost the very southern tip of Vietnam to the Northern part. When we got to Hanoi there was a car waiting to take us to our hotel called The Rising Dragon Villa. Even though our room was under $30 a night they had arranged for our airport pick up which was a nice treat since the ride was nearly an hour to the main part of the city where we would be staying. The price of the cab wasn't included in the room but we found it was helpful when entering into a new city to have a car waiting to snag us up, so long as the fair was uh, fair.

Airport Travel Tips

144

Be sure to know what you can and can't bring on a flight so you don't have to avoid throwing things out that you would much rather keep. There are, of course, certain advantages to flying with limited luggage and having a carry-on bag; quick check in, not having to wait for your bags at your destination, less chance of losing personal belongings, someone messing with your stuff. But you should consider what you are bringing to the airport, and if you are traveling with knives and sharp objects like us, you don't have much choice but to check your bag, or donate your knives in one city and buy a cheap one in the next.

Also, if you have large liquids such as sunscreen (which I advise you buy ahead of time as it is expensive in Vietnam and other similar countries), you will either need to check your bag or a great trick is to portion it up into smaller containers so it is under the legal flying limit.

Getting a cab from the major airports is easy but always make sure you have the name of the place you are going written down so the driver can easily understand your destination. To make things even easier, reach out to the hotel you are staying at and see if they will send someone to pick you up. It may cost you a few extra bucks but having a driver who knows where to go is always a big bonus, especially after an exhausting day of travel.

The drive into Hanoi was scenic with its old and partially run down buildings of varying blues, reds and greens mixed in with more subtle colors all stacked up next to one another, the city had a lot of character and while it wasn't as lively and modern as Ho Chi Minh, it had a classier and more historic feel to it, I could even notice the French architectural influences in a lot of the buildings.

As we got closer and closer I noticed what seemed like an endless amount of Karaoke bars, 'We are in for a treat', I thought, though only half joking to myself as I hadn't had much karaoke experience, even if I did start a rock band with my brother and sister when I was ten. When we got into the main part of town, it was interesting to see just how different it was from Ho Chi Minh city. While they had the usual crowded streets complete with street vendors, food stalls, shops selling all sorts of goodies and motorbikes galore, the structure of the town, with its winding streets and compressed crowds, had quite a different energy than we had experienced down South. We were staying in what was called "Old City," a name that couldn't be more fitting, you could feel it's long standing history with each passing block.

When we arrived at the hotel, which was highly ranked and by far the nicest place we had booked to stay, we asked to see our $30 a night room. They took us right up and when we walked in we knew we had found a much better spot than the hotel in Ho Chi Minh. The room was huge, luxurious, no toilet/shower combination where the shower is just a spout from the wall, where when you wash yourself you end up washing the rest of the bathroom by accident. Nope, not here! There was an actual shower with glass door and everything, two windows peering out into the busy street below, good counter space, there was even a refrigerator in our room. At that point we made sure that every place we stayed at had a fridge, for us it was necessary, and boy did we pack the crap out of the minute we got in.

Tips for Hotel Rooms

Always ask to see your room before committing to it. Usually everything is okay but it never hurts to see the room and make sure it is to your liking. Also, if there is something missing such as a fridge or hot water heater it never hurts to ask if they can bring it to your room. Asking doesn't cost anything, worst case they say no and you are no lesser off than you were.

After we unpacked and relaxed for a few minutes it was time for us to hit the streets. We had initially planned to stay in Hanoi for a few days, then head to Halong Bay, then Sapa, and then go down the coast, but I wasn't feeling 100% and as much as we wanted to get to Sapa, a beautiful region way up south famous for it's sprawling hills lined with rice paddies, we realized it was better to relax, recharge and focus on being present and enjoying where ever we were at the moment. The 8-hour train ride each way to Sapa at first seemed fun and romantic, but now, being accustomed to the sweltering heat, we knew the train ride would leave us burnt out. We decided to stay a few extra days in Hanoi, take things slowly and not trying to cram everything into such a short amount of time.

When you're traveling, and so far from home, often it seems logical to see and do and really cram in as much as you humanly can, not knowing when you might make it back to the other side of the world. But sometimes it becomes too much, and often takes you away from being present and enjoying any one thing. We've found, from years of travel, that staying local, exploring even just one, or a few cities, can lead to enough of an adventure and really help you get to understand the culture better, not just hit the touristy hot spots.

On our way out of the hotel we asked the front desk if there were any good food markets we could go to and the concierge pointed us in the right direction. We didn't have a workable cellphone or internet outside of the hotel, but we were able to plug the destination into the map on our phone and follow along the route.

Having a clear destination in hand, open to wherever the journey might lead us, we went out to explore yet another new city. As we walked along the busy streets we noticed, like Ho Chi Minh, most of the walking would be done in the street and not on the already crowded sidewalks, where there were a lot of people, all minding their own business, going about their day.

As we walked we started to see that there were a bunch of people sitting on very small and blue or red colored stools, about a foot off the ground, maybe less, all eating a large bowl of noodle soup with some sort of pastry in it. We found the source—a man sitting behind probably the biggest pot of steaming soup that I had ever seen, furiously working away, adding some fresh rice noodles to a pot of boiling water, ladling the clear and fragrant broth into a large bowl crammed with rice noodles, right before adding in thinly sliced beef and sprinkling chopped up green onions on top and handing it to the hungry locals, patiently sitting on the barely above ground stools, while someone else topped it with a few savory pastries that looked like long thin fried donuts made out of wheat flour.

I could tell that Josh wanted to try some and so I urged him to order a bowl. Sometimes I can tell he feels a little guilty being able to eat any deliciousness that he sees, knowing that I usually can't join in, but I always encourage him to try anything that looks good, so long as it seems hygienically safe. We sat down and he got Hanoi's famous dish, Pho Bo (Beef noodle soup) while carrying a large grin on his face. He happily slurped away, while I took in the sights and slew of people and motorbikes whizzing ever so closely by the street side "restaurant". The bowl of soup looked delicious, and was gluten free for that matter, but it of course had meat in it and was made from a bone broth, so I wouldn't be eating any, though it wouldn't make me sick if I did. Josh said the Pho, which only set him back $1, was mind blowingly delicious, the warm and soothing aromatic broth, chewy rice noodles to soak in all the flavor and tender, barely poached beef, made for the perfect balance in what was his favorite soup of all time. Whereas the Pho in Ho Chi Minh came with a large side fresh greens to go in, in Hanoi it came fully loaded as is, without much greens, and you could add in some flavorful condiments like chili and fish sauce if you'd like.

When I was dating in past relationships, when someone would eat something that I could not consume I would feel left out or sometimes even less. than. Over time I have truly learned how to appreciate food from smelling it and seeing someone else enjoy it, it may sound strange, but it's a good feeling seeing someone you love happily chomping down on a delicious meal. Besides, from my travels I have learned the importance of bringing along snacks to munch on or stocking up on fresh fruit along the way while the person that I was with ate so I could at least share in the edible experience.

Once Josh finished the soup we attempted to find a pharmacy on our path towards the market. I was in need of some serious menstrual pain help and hoped to find some Midol or a natural remedy such as turmeric pills to help with cramping but after much wandering we turned up with little luck. It was at that moment that I realized for as much stuff as I brought to make sure I was set in the health and food department of travels, I had forgotten about that one, so important, area.

We kept on searching for the market we had heard about but as we walked past the dot on the map we came upon an opening to a huge lake surrounded by a paved path with locals peacefully walking, or jogging, along it. It was a beautifully calm and serene lake with an ancient, four tired, semi open structure in the middle of the massive body of water.

We walked along it, hand in hand, in search of any sign of the grocery store. Trying desperately to find the physical location of the dot on the map, we seemed to walk right by where it said it was but didn't mind as it was such a beautiful day. It's easy when you are in a new place to get lost and turned upside down not realizing quite where you are because there is so much to take in around you. We walked so far passed the dot on the map, hoping the directions were off and that we might stumble upon the market as if by magic, but somehow ended up in what felt like another country as we walked into a really high end mall with Versace, Gucci and other top end retailers. I was starting to feel like I was back at home in the states, almost as if we'd walked into a parallel dimension or some invisible time portal, it was extremely odd going from this majestic historic town center to a modern luxury mall as we struggled to find our planned destination.

After a much needed bathroom break we managed to find the exit to the shopping labyrinth we had entered and on our way out of the mall we saw a bride and groom to be taking their wedding photos. Taking in such a common ritual from back home in another country was really interesting. On the one hand, it was really cute to see the couple all dressed up and posing for pictures, but on the other, from my perspective I can't say I got the impression that they were in love. That being said, the more time we spent in Vietnam, the more we understood that showing public affection wasn't necessarily welcomed with open arms. Not to say we had a problem with this, as every culture has their own culture norms, it did take some time to adjust to the fact that even holding Josh's hand as we walked down the street felt somehow taboo and out of place.

We walked back down the same street near the lake to try and find the grocery store before finally giving up and, upon a small inclination, we noticed that there was an alleyway leading to a large parking lot that was right by the dot on the map claiming to be the grocery store. When we followed the small road towards the back of the building we noticed that there was a large amount of motorbikes parked alongside one another and to the right of that we saw an opening to... the grocery store, score! It's no wonder we completely missed it the first few times we walked by, the whole time we were searching for a sign and not thinking beyond our understanding of how things were back home.

Upon entering what we now felt like was our mini food mecca, we saw an open, and slightly modernized, grocery store with a decently sized produce section to our left, standard isles filled with pantry items amongst other things to our right, and stairs leading up to a second floor. As we meandered through the produce section we quickly realized that it was not much to write home about, the prices were high, the quality was sub par at best, but we were not here for produce, as we left that to the local markets, no, we wanted to find a gas can for the burner (considering we could not fly with them - highly illegal and explosive) and some other cooking essentials. Besides, checking out random markets in new places is one of our favorite things to do, finding new ingredients and treats we have never seen, I guess for us it's like shoe shopping for sneaker heads. Another bonus for me is that in some of the bigger and more commercialized markets I can often find translated ingredients listed on the back of some of the products that might be exclusively in Vietnamese at the local markets. Yay for ingredient lists!

After about twenty minutes of searching we came up short on finding a gas canister for the burner but one thing I did find that I thought to be interesting was lotus seed chips, made from nothing but lotus seeds and oil. They were certainly more expensive than a regular bag of chips but they looked interesting, I was intrigued and decided to buy a pack.

When we left the grocery store we decided to take a few things we had bought and have a little romantic mini picnic by the lake. Some peanut butter, raisins, lotus seeds and an apple, plus some hand wipes, seemed like the perfect snack. When we opened the lotus seeds and gave them a taste the first thing I noticed was how crunchy they were. The second thing I noticed was that they were super sweet, and third thing that I noticed was that they were at the moment the best thing I had ever had! They tasted just like shortbread cookies, or more like those nilla wafers I used to love as a kid, I was in heaven. If only they weren't so expensive I would have bought a lot more. Expensive for even the American dollar at least, for the bag costed $10.

After our picnic, we headed to one of the local outdoor produce markets to buy some food for the upcoming days, we knew that once we had a gas canister our hotel room would transform into a full-on kitchen, but for the moment we could at least make some raw food. We found some local outdoor vendors selling fresh rice noodles, a colorful array of fresh produce, exotic fruits, tofu and meat of all cuts and sizes. We picked up all that we could carry, colorful vegetables, vibrantly smelling fruits, and herbs, all for a whopping $5, and headed back to the hotel to get some much-needed rest.

Market Shopping Tips
As we mentioned earlier, local market shopping can be a bit intimidating, but it is absolutely one of the best way to get a simple taste of local life as well as dirt cheap prices. Learning a few key phrases can go

a long way. Things like "how much does this cost?" or "that price is too high," can really help you navigate the local language. A great part about shopping at local markets is that you usually know what you are buying, Even if you don't know the translation, you see the ingredient and you pick out how much you want, it's a simple and safe way to get fresh food.

Don't be afraid to say "that is too much," and walk away. Not all the people selling food on the street are friendly, most people are, but you will find a mix. We found that it was best to stick to buying from someone that is helpful. If you try to buy from someone and they wave you away or seem uninterested, do not be afraid to go to another vendor. Typically you'll find multiple people selling an array of the same stuff with small differences in quality, variety and price. In Vietnam you'll find fresh produce being sold everywhere, even on moving carts, it's lovely.

The next day we spent the bulk of our time exploring the area, checking out the streets, the food, and of course searching for a gas canister so that we could cook. We found that the same market we went to the night before to buy some produce was far busier and lively during the day, a common thing especially early mornings as it's typical for locals to shop daily for produce. We found a kitchen supply area, did some bargaining and ended up with three more gas canisters plus a new large pot we could use to make soups, costing a total of $6. We had been in Vietnam nearly a week and already it was hard to not want to move there and create a simple life, everything was so inexpensive! Tempting, but unlikely.

At that point, seeing Josh enjoy such a plethora of delicious warm bowls of soup, I was craving a big bowl of my own. The one they served at the Homestay looked too good, it had me on soup envy, and we felt confident between the two of us that we could create a very similar version minus the fish. We bought cabbage, tomatoes, pineapples, garlic, onions and turmeric as well as fresh rice noodles. After spending some time buying a few other things at the market, including a bad ass knife for $1, we brought the food home and began cooking.

Making soup, in a hotel of all places, might seem a bit absurd, and for that matter it may have been, but the process of making soup is truly a relaxing feat. One thing that I have come to discover about the art of soup making is that it can be as simple or complex as you want it to be. By focusing on the fresh ingredients you can really pull out their flavors and add it to the broth.

We filled our pan with some cold water and began adding in the chopped up veggies and spices we had. From the start we placed in one tomato cut up into small pieces, some minced up garlic and turmeric, chopped onions, half of an apple and a pinch of salt. When making a soup you don't want to add to much salt until the very end as when the soup boils down the salt will concentrate. At this point we let the water come to a boil and turned the burner down to a simmer to let the veggies and spices really infuse into the broth.

After about ten minutes we started tasting the broth to see how the flavors were talking together in one giant conversation of deliciousness. The flavor was light and delicate so we kept letting it cook down. We tossed in the cabbage after another 10 minutes and let it simmer down more. Once the broth was too our liking, we added in some more salt to bring out the flavors and served the soup with some fresh rice noodles and some fresh chili we had grabbed at the market.

All in all it was a simple and satisfying meal that really comforted my belly and made me feel warm and at peace. Whether or not you have the audacity to whip up a soup while traveling, just know that as exciting as it is to try out fresh food on the street, having access to the ingredients of a culture that is new to you is equally, if not more, exciting, and using the ingredients in a simple way can leave you and your belly fully satisfied.

After our soup we took a nice walk, something we love to do after every meal to help our digestion get it's groove on, and then plopped our butts into bed. All in all, we had a lovely day exploring Hanoi and decided to head off into dream land early because we had some exciting plans the following day. Josh had contacted another one of his Youtube fans who was eager to show us around Hanoi as Kelly had in Saigon, and while they did help keep me safe in the eating department, I had my first taste of real danger on a scooter.

Chapter 13:

Not the Safest Way to Get Around

The next morning we woke up and hit the breakfast area which we had missed the day before on account of sleeping in a little too late. We were shocked to find just how much free food they offered here, they had an entire list of American and Vietnamese breakfast classics like noodle soup, pancakes, eggs, and French toast as well as a bountiful buffet. For me, while I didn't have many options, there was a ton of fruit; dragon fruit, pineapple and melons galore. I politely asked if they could cut me up some fresh fruit on a plastic cutting board to avoid cross contamination and to my surprise they happily said yes. Sure I could have easily made my own fruit parfait in the hotel room with what we had bought but there is truly something special about these little magic moments.

Safe Food Eating Tip

It is perfectly okay to ask for something a little more personalized if you are offered a free buffet at your hotel or homestay. If they offer fruit, don't be afraid to even ask them for a whole uncut fruit. Show your allergy card and let them know why you are asking. You deserve a free breakfast like everyone else and even if it is only fruit you are entitled to your breakfast. Pretty much everywhere we went everyone was very helpful and willing to help out. People in Vietnam generally take food very seriously, it is a huge part of their culture, and while there will always people that get annoyed, and others that simply don't understand, you are a paying guest and the Hotel's number one priority is to make you feel taken care of, and eating a meal is top of the importance list for most.

After breakfast, we headed out back into town to wander the streets, checking out clothes and food. Josh spotted this dish a bunch of locals were eating that looked really unique. It was called Banh Trang Tron, it's a common snack made of rice paper cut up in thin strips, mixed with a hard-boiled quail egg, some vegetables, a few types of Vietnamese beef jerky that looked hardly anything like the one we have back in the states, all tossed in a spicy sauce that softens the noodles and makes them chewy.

Josh told me the dish was absolutely amazing and unlike anything he had ever eaten although I could see the tears running down his eyes as he fought hard to handle the heat of that chili sauce. It was precious and hilarious and reminded me of one of our first dates at Union Pool in Brooklyn where we shared habanero salsa tacos. I had ordered two tacos extra spicy and he, probably wanting to impress me, ordered the same. He took the tiniest of bites, sweating, breathing heavy, eating so slowly, trying to show me that he could handle the heat, it was adorable. Luckily for me, while he can't always handle the food's heat, he can always, well usually, handle mine.

After a little exploring we met up with Josh's fan. As she rolled up on her motorbike we noticed it was not one but three girls; Ha`ng, Bi'ch, and Kim-Ly, they all had similar short brown hair, bangs partially covering their eyes, all around 18 years old, all bright eyed and cheery. Within minutes of greeting us they politely asked us in a broken english to get on the back of their motorbikes so they could take us on a little tour of the town.

In Ho Chi Minh city, though I was a bit nervous getting on a motorbike, I trusted the older, more experienced drivers, who seemed to taxi people back and forth as a profession, but with these girls, I must admit, I was a little unsure. I shot Josh an uneasy look, he opened up a quick smile and after a moment of hesitation, I said screw it and we jumped on the back before speeding off to, where, we didn't know.

Within 5 minutes of cruising my driver, Kim-Ly, seemed to lose the rest of the crew. My heart was starting to race, I had no phone incase I lost Josh, if something happened to us he would have no way of knowing, and her steering wasn't exactly the most, uh, controlled. Weaving from left to right, jam packed with what felt like thousands of other eager riders, as I held onto her for dear life, she nearly smacked us into a truck all the while laughing and talking the whole way through like it was totally normal.

I won't lie, I was freaking terrified and wondered for a brief second if I would ever see my boo again, but all in all I was hopeful that we had made it this far through our trip with no issues and that nothing would happen now. Within what felt like being an inch between life and death, I couldn't help but think about how grateful, sickness or not, I was to have gone on this trip in the first place

Having a positive outlook is important in any situation, especially while traveling, you always want to be smart and safe in an unknown place but sometimes you are going to get yourself into risky situations and keeping your head up and your thoughts good always helps me on the road.

After we made a mad dash out of the busy Hanoi streets we finally found everyone else and buzzed on for another ten minutes until we finally found out way in the outskirts of the city by some large monuments. Figuring as it was our first time in Vietnam they wanted to show us some of the classic touristy spots, even if we had not asked. The first stop was Ho Chi Minh's grave site, a major touristy attraction. Ho Chi Minh was the famous general that the southern city is named after. It was beautiful, unlike any area of a town I had ever seen, the colors were so vibrant and it felt as though we had been transported to another time.

After showing us around, Ha`ng, who seemed like the cheerful and sweet leader of the pack said that they were eager to show us some of the food in Hanoi which was honestly a relief because we had all had enough of the touristy stuff. They kept telling us how much they loved to try new food, and expressed how much they loved watching Josh's YouTube show to learn about other cultures. It was so sweet and inspiring to see the way they took so much from his show and how they had this connection to Josh and learning how to cook from a million miles away

Before we got back on their bikes, Josh, who could tell I felt a bit unsafe riding with the same girl again, happily traded bikes with me, and after a short motorbike ride they took us to a main strip in Hanoi filled with food vendors. We walked and walked until we found a place that had another famous Vietnamese dish, Green Papaya salad. The green papaya was first shaved razor thin into little noodle like strips, it was then typically mixed with some fresh herbs, cooked ground pork, peanuts and tossed with a lime and fish sauce dressing. It looked delicious, and for the first time during the trip I felt like I wanted to try and see if the vendor was open to altering her recipe in favor of one that I could eat. One of the girls translated for me to see what the vendor could do. As it turns out she was able to make it without the pork but not without the fish sauce because the dressing was pre-made. In lieu of the good company, and me wanting to try it because papaya salad was one of my favorites, I ordered a small plate to try. It was the rule I had always had since I stopped eating meat, though it hardly ever happened, if I ever craved something that was safe on my allergy list but not vegan, I would not deprive myself.

Unfortunately, after one small bite, I quickly scrunched my face in disapproval, making everyone laugh, Josh included. Fish sauce, as it turns out, was not for me. I quickly ran to the bathroom to spit out the food and rinsed my mouth with some bottled water to get the fishy taste out of my mouth, yuck! But no matter, I learned that I still didn't like eating animal products, it was all good, I enjoyed spending time with everyone while they ate their papaya salads all while remembering why I stopped enjoying animal products in the first place.

After everyone finished the papaya salad which I was told was absolutely refreshing and delicious, Josh mentioned to me that he really wanted to try grilled pigeon and snails but was unsure of the best place to order it. Seeing as how we were hanging out with some locals we figured they would help point us in the direction of something safe. They mentioned that they too wanted to eat snail and happily took us to their favorite spot.

Half expecting to walk into a restaurant, half just going with the flow, we weren't all that surprised to find out that the place they took us to was a street stall, set with tiny chairs and tables set up next to an older Vietnamese woman who had a big of fresh snails, all ready to be cooked up. The snails, believe it or not, looked great and brought me right back to Culinary school where I used to enjoy my share of the little chewy critters. I sat there, completely relaxed, taking in the scene playing out before me as the group ate their steamed snails that they took out of the shell with a small metal tool and dipped it into a chili garlic fish dip. I could hardly believe how much I used to enjoy snails, remembering all the times I used to eat them drenched in butter with herbs and white wine, I sat in amazement thinking about how much my palate had changed since I stopped eating animal products.

After all of the little snails were eaten up, we walked a bit more and stumbled upon an interesting vendor who had a special pastry rolled with coconut flakes and some sort of crispy palm sugar candy that looked divine. I couldn't try the treat the man was serving but I noticed that the palm sugar candy was in a separate sealed packet and after one of the girls helped me translate to the street vendor we found out that it was safe, score! We bought some of the intriguing candy, he was happy to sell it to us without the rest of the treat, it was crispy, sweet and delicious, a unique texture that was a lot lighter than most of the treats I had had before. Even though I wasn't able to enjoy the entire dessert, it was nice to know that some street vendors were willing to customize something or sell you a part of a dish if you asked politely (or had the help of a local to guid the way).

I was happy to tag along as Josh and the girls had their filling of delicious street food, having eaten a few hours before was a lifesaver, but seeing as how it was dessert and that I had not been able to eat much on our little street food adventure Josh insisted that we find a place that I could eat too, he is always so considerate in that way. Being inclusive is something that I encourage in relationships, finding ways to enjoy meals together, ways to empower each other through the process of sharing really helps build your bond. Ultimately, it's not just about what you eat, but how you eat it and the experience you create with the people that you care about the most.

They took us to their favorite dessert spot where, as luck would have it, everything was safe for me. They reintroduced us to a dessert that we recognized from our eating adventure with Kelly in Ho Chi Minh, *Che,* the dessert comprised of different jellies, coconut milk and crushed ice. This place had a full menu of sweet and chewy goodness and a ton of interesting options to choose from.

We ordered 5 different things and went to town. Oh my god, it was so sweet, yet so delicious. I could eat all the different treats we had ordered, the different jelly like textures mixed with candied fruits, crushed ice and fresh coconut milk, heaven in my mouth. Again, it is important to make sure the ice is safe but we found that asking if the ice was made from mineral water was always a good way to ensure that the ice was safe, especially if it wasn't in the circular shape we had been told to watch for. Often times vendors would point to a clean bottle of water to let us know that they made their ice from a proper source.

We ate and ate, I felt like I couldn't stop, even debated getting more except after a while of munching I started to feel all the sugar on my teeth and knew I had to put my spoon down. Somehow, I have developed a sensitivity to certain sugars since eating cleaner and I can feel when there is processed sugar in foods. It's not something I'd eat everyday but it is a real treat from time to time. Besides, finding something, anything, that is cold, crunchy, creamy and sweet that doesn't have dairy in it is always a win for me.

After saying our goodbyes and thanking the girls for showing us around, we headed back early that night to get some much-needed rest, chatting about how fun, and terrifying, it was riding on the motorbikes with the girls. When we got back to our room we busted out some of the palm sugar candies we had bought from the vendor and made this crazy delicious treat where we wrapped the candies in rice paper with peanut butter and watermelon. Ridiculous? Maybe. Delicious? Oh yeah! I guess we still had a little sugar craving to fulfill in the comforts of our own hotel. Overall, it was a great day. I was feeling much better in Hanoi, hardly noticed any issues with the heat or my body, my hormones seemed in check, I felt fresh, hydrated and calm. Things were starting to look up, it was starting to look like I could beat this thing and have a great trip after all. A little hope was all I needed to be reminded of why we took this journey in the first place.

Chapter 14:

Part Time Tourists

The next morning, we talked to the concierge about taking a boat tour to Halong bay and after a train to Da Nang. They informed us that the train to the center of the country was 18 hours long while the Halong Bay boat trip could be a two or three-night cruise. We were told that taking the train could be a fun, though arduous journey. You could get a sleeper which would replace the need for a hotel for the night, but it was certainly a long journey. We decided to sleep on it and see how we felt as the day's passed.

After some back and forth, the plan, we decided, was to focus on planning our trip to Halong Bay, an area said to be famous for being surrounded by hundreds of beautiful islands and blue water for days, where you could book a trip on a boat with a guided tour which included food, room, transportation and all. We had planned to head to the middle of the country after our boat trip but at the moment we were focused on finding the right trip, one where I could safely eat the food, as we decided it was best to not attempt to cook with our little burner, on a boat, in the middle of the ocean… Not exactly safe, though I must admit, what fun that would have been.

It took some time to decide on the right boat for us, but after some time talking to the hotel travel guide, Josh and I took one last look at the pamphlets and decided to pick the imperial cruise ship, it was a bit more expensive compared to our other options, but it looked nice and we wanted to make sure that the food would be safe for me to eat. This would be one of the few touristy things that we did on the trip but we were told it was the only way to see Halong Bay and it seemed like a lot of fun. Sure, we would have loved to take out our own personal boat, but in Halong Bay, you have to go with what they have set up for you.

The hotel travel guide, Fern, called the ship to make sure that they could safely handle my food allergies, and when they seemed the most confident we jumped on the chance to cruise the open waters for a few days, even if we were packed in with other tourists and stuck to a schedule.

In the end we chose the cruise for two nights and three days as we heard that often times the one night two day cruises left you feeling like you were spending most of your time traveling to get to the dang boat and once you got there the whole trip was pretty much over. Sometimes when you are forced to make a decision while traveling, you simply have to trust your gut.

The next morning we would be picked up early on a shuttle bus and taken to the boats, so we used our last day in Hanoi as a chance to get some last exploring in as well as prep for the upcoming days. We made sure to buy fresh veggies and prepare some food in the event that I needed something along the journey, even though we were told the boat could cook for me safely, I wanted to have some backup provisions.

During lunch, Josh stopped at a small spot on the street and ordered a dish that neither of us even knew existed. Pho Xao, as it turns out, is basically a stir-fried version of Pho where the rice noodles are fried in a sauce mixed with beef and topped with bean sprouts. He absolutely loved it and insisted that we create a Jaquy version with some of the ingredients we had bought.

When we got back to the hotel we did our best to recreate this street food delight with sautéd rice noodles, mushrooms and mung beans in a savory garlic sauce. Not only was it absolutely delicious, but luckily we made enough to have leftovers for the trek the next day along with some fresh slaw and steamed veggies that we could dip in our master chili sauce. I have to say, as much as I got envious of all the epic food that Josh was eating, even cooking the simplest of meals in a foreign country, especially one like Vietnam that has such great produce, for so cheap, was always such a delight. I was continually amazed by how good the food tasted, even when we simply steamed some veggies with salt and chili, it somehow tasted exotic and unique.

Cooking With Gas Tip

While not everyone is going to be as thrifty, and daring, as we were when cooking on the road, if you don't feel comfortable using a gas stove, you can always buy, or bring a small portable electric stove to heat food up. For around $20 you can pick a small single burner up and bring it around in your suitcase. There are also great little mini steamers and slow cookers you can find online that can help you along the way too.

That night, after we finished cooking, we got some much needed rest for what we knew would be a long, though exciting, day ahead of us.

In the morning we snagged some breakfast at the hotel and were picked up by a shuttle bus that went from hotel to hotel grabbing passengers who would be part of our trip. Transportation was certainly my least favorite part and I found that I was getting carsick as the car kept stopping every few minutes to pick up more people. Josh reminded me to focus on looking outside and drinking as much water as possible which did seem to help.

The group was a mixed bag; some college students, a few older couples, two families, a handful of backpackers around our age, all very kind, excited, and laid back. All was going well until we arrived at our last destination to pick up the final family. When our tour tour guide got off to grab them it seemed that he was having some problems with them as he said they only booked for six people, but were actually ten when we arrived at their hotel, little kids included. The family acted as though it was no big deal and sort of shoved their way onto the bus. Four screaming little kids and all… great, just our luck.

When we finally got to the Halong Bay dock there were hundreds of other people all in chaos trying to find their tour groups and get to their boats. We were given a ticket and told that if we lost it we would not be getting onto the boat without buying another and that while it was originally included in the price of the trip, a replacement was very expensive. While we waited around we struck up a conversation with a sweet Australian family. Aja, a naturally beautiful and dark skinned woman who was part Indian, had an effortless about her kindness, and a welcoming nature that made me feel right at home. Her son, Demetri, who was around ten years old, was super sweet, albeit a little shy, which wasn't a surprise considering he was one of the few children in a sea of adults.

When we were introduced to Aja's husband, Michael, at first I was a little thrown off. Having a wife so sweet it came to a bit of surprise when he was so standoffish and quiet. He looked uncomfortable or like he wasn't feeling well, but I wasn't quite sure.

It wasn't until I asked to go to the bathroom before getting onto the boat that I found out why Michael was acting the way he was. As he recapped the story, he and his family had been traveling the week before in Malaysia and he had eaten something that gave him bad food poisoning, he hadn't kept any food down at all for the past two days, he said it was miserable and he couldn't wait to get back to eating again because he knew how could the food in Vietnam was. I gave him some tips on how to stay hydrated and get his body back into proper working order and as we spoke I came to find he was just as sweet and friendly as his wife.

We took a small motor boat that shuttled us out to our main boat in the middle of the bay. All of the boats in Halong bay looked practically the same with their big white sails which seemed a bit odd at first as there was nothing on the bay but blue water, an endless sea of variously shaped and sized islands and the boats. The boat, once we got on it, was quite spacious and clean, holding around 30 to 40 people plus a sizable crew.

When we saw our room, it kind of blew us away, it had everything we could need in such a small package. Large bed, full shower and bathroom, some space for our clothing, and huge windows looking out onto the water. It was nice for a boat, though I didn't have much experience staying on boats, so I suppose it was perfectly normal.

After we dropped our stuff off we were asked to lunch which I assumed at first would be difficult because it takes a few times to explain to a team and chef how to properly handle Celiac disease and my food allergies. This was my first time on a boat in Vietnam let alone my first time in a structured tour group since I was 16 when I took a cruise with my mom to the tropics. At the time I swore up and down that I would never do that again because it made me feel claustrophobic. Sure I had some fears, and sure, the boat tour may have been more touristy, but we already had such a great and authentic local experience over the past two weeks that we kind of wanted to see what it would be like from the other side.

Regardless of what they said when we called in and asked about the food, I had to be extra careful eating as I didn't want to ruin the rest of the trip. Even if they claimed on the phone that they could handle my restrictions safely, and that they had experience with it, we made sure to go over everything with the chef. We did have extra food for me, not enough to last the whole trip, but to get us through a day or so, but I hoped we would not have to use it.

Surprisingly they were extremely attentive, they said they could accommodate everything and make special food that would be safe for me. At first I was surprised but I suppose one benefit of doing something touristy is that they have more general experience with tourists, whereas random street carts may have no clue. As lunch came out I was amazed, the food just didn't stop coming, fresh rice, steamed veggies, sautéed greens, tofu, fried fish, meat, it went on and on and on. The food I ate was mostly steamed veggies, rice and fresh fruits but I brought my magic bottle sauce that had fresh turmeric, vinegar, lime juice, garlic and chilies. The master sauce helped but regardless everything was fresh and delicious. None of the food on the boat looked much like authentic Vietnamese food but the presentation and sheer volume of dishes was enough to make anyone, Josh included, satisfied.

After lunch, we were taken to a beautiful cave on one of the islands to walk around and take some pictures. Halong Bay is made up of hundreds of small blue rock islands with lush green tops surrounded by beautiful clear blue waters. All the boats taking tourists around Halong Bay are pretty similar as we had come to see, all painted white with big sails just for show. We found out that the reason the boats all had to look the same and be painted white was because of a law passed years ago, for safety, due to some previous issues with pirates, yes, you read that right, real pirates! But nothing to worry about of course, or so we were told…

After the cave visit we went on a tandem kayak for the two of us where we had nearly an hour to paddle around. On the one hand, it was the most majestically beautiful kayak ride I had ever taken; the clear blue skies, the vibrant water, fresh air, outside of the city, blowing in our face… But on the other hand, where we took out the kayak, it was on a tiny floating village that was quite dirty, there was trash floating all over the place. It made me sad that there was so much disregard for preserving the natural way of things, honestly it was kind of disgusting getting splashed by the dirty water filled of candy wrappers and garbage, but it was still fun and we made the most of it. Besides, going into it we had heard stories of the trash issues so it's not like we were totally surprised.

When we got back on the boat, there was a huge dinner of fried fish, chicken, veggies, rice and more veggies for me, they even carved a bird out of carrots and some fruits. I had all the food I could imagine, I felt so loved and cared for! It was nuts… After dinner, there was karaoke, ah yes, now all of those signs in Hanoi were starting to make sense. Little did I know just how much the Vietnamese people love their karaoke. One of the crew members began singing a Vietnamese song with an incredible amount of passion, I swear he could have gone on that show American Idol and slayed, even if he didn't have the greatest voice.

After singing his song and attempting, with virtually no luck, to wrangle up any of the guests on the boat to jump on the mic he saw Josh looking wide eyed and called him over to pick a song. He must have known or seen how magnetic Josh looked to do some singing, because within a few moments he had him serenading the entire boat, singing such classics as "Hotel California" and Bob Marley's "Three Little Birds." It was the best thing I had ever seen and the entire boat was thrilled and loving it! It lit up my heart to see him slaying the crowd and having such a good time, I kept telling myself that's my boo!

After karaoke, we were ready for some fresh air so we headed to the roof, it was a most beautiful night, it seemed like the stars were shining extra bright just for us that night. Some people were squid fishing, using flash lights in the near pitch dark with no luck, others chatted away, but not Josh. Oh no, Josh had the idea to entertain some of the guests with some light painting. If you've never light painted before, it's pretty awesome. Basically, you take a camera in the pitch dark and set the exposure to stay open for a long period of time. What this does is that it allows the camera to capture any light coming in and if you take a flash light you can actually "paint" and draw on the picture. If you still don't get what it's all about, google "light painting," you'll be amazed.

After Josh started drawing in the air with the light on his phone, some of the other members of the tour starting walking over, intrigued by what they were seeing, and pretty soon just about everyone on the boat was loving it, watching with great attention, joining in to the fun.

We met two older Irish women in their 80's, Selma and Carol, who said that every year since Selma had lost her husband they took a trip to another part of the world, to have fun and remember how wonderful life is. They were both so charming and wise, it made me think of my mom and how I wished that she would do the same—take adventures and remember that life is a blessing and every day is meant to explore something new.

The next morning I awoke to nothing but stillness. Looking out our cabin window I saw the bright blue sky, vibrant and alive as the sun peeked its way over the horizon. We were sailing around the bay ever so gently, I could hardly tell if we were moving or if my mind was playing tricks on me.

When I got to the deck there was a big breakfast prepared but seeing as how my only option was fruit I made sure to have my trusty protein powder mixture ready to go. A little hot water and a bowl and I was set to head off on our next adventure, a pearl farm.

I was never really into fancy jewelry but I thought seeing the process of making pearls would be interesting and for that matter it really was. They showed us how they implant these tiny basic pearls into the oysters and how they harvest them months later to create a beautiful pearl from the original implant, I had no idea that was how the process went. I did however want to up my Julia Child game and was hoping to buy some pearls, but unfortunately, they were extremely expensive so I figured it was best to keep looking and hope that the right pearls would present themselves to me at the right time.

After the pearl farm I was getting super excited because I knew that we would have one night on Cat Ba island, a really secluded and romantic looking island, off of the ship, to spend our final time during our adventure at sea. During our mini boat trip, we had become close to the Australian couple, sharing life stories, bonding over meals, and filling them in on our reason for taking the trip and how we would be writing a book about the journey once it was over. As it turns out, when we were saying our goodbye's, Michael, the father, said that our story inspired him to take a stab at a lifelong passion of his that he never got around to doing. He had always wanted to write a book and said talking to us helped him work up the courage. Hearing that was truly amazing, life is funny and beautiful in that way, you never know who you might inspire when you are following your own journey.

Not everyone on our trip, the Australian family included, had signed up for the extra night on Cat Ba Island. As it turns out we would be getting off our big boat and onto a smaller boat with other travelers we had yet to meet to head to the Island. It was a nice change of pace but it also meant I had a new crew that I had to re-explain all of my allergies to.

During the ride the crew did their best to understand what I could not eat but they kept confusing wheat with rice which made them uneasy as they pretty much eat rice with everything. Between me trying to explain to them how I could not eat certain foods, them getting confused, the hot sun pulsating overhead, the intense humidity, and big waves that seemed to mercilessly beat the tiny boat down like a bully on the playground, I was starting to feel sea sick and nauseous. It seemed like the closer they said we were to arriving at the island the farther that island felt, like a mirage of water you desperately want to drink to fulfill that immense thirst, always just out of reach. I guess that's what sea sickness does to me.

Trying to beat the motion sickness I sat at the front of the boat in hopes that it would help balance me out as we sailed through the islands, trying different breathing exercises to center myself, but it was really rough. I was feeling like a dried-up piece of fruit being peeled off the floor, flapping in the wind, bouncing upside down, feeling like my insides were about to come up.

When we finally arrived at Cat Ba island, it was breathtaking, like a picture out of Natural Geographic spread, one of those shots that makes you think there is no way this is actually what it looks like in real person, my brain could hardly process how majestically beautiful and picturesque it was, but at the same time it was taking all of my energy to stay focused on my simple breathing techniques so as to not spew my guts all over the place like a freshman in college who just arrived at their first keg party.

Once we got on to the island and waited to receive our room assignments while sitting at a table in the dining area, which by the way felt, in my contorted state, like we were at Hogwarts just waiting to see where the sorting hat would place us, I couldn't help but hope the room we booked really had air conditioning in it. From the looks of it the bungalows were small and they seemed rather primitive. All I wanted to do, in the wake of the excessive heat, was jack that air conditioning machine up to full blast and crash into bed on solid ground, a bed that wasn't rocking up and down like a pogo stick.

Our room was a small bungalow with a full-sized bed, a humble (primitive) shower and air-conditioning (thank heavens!) with a beautiful view of the bay and a cozy porch with two wooden chairs and a small table on it. Big score for the air conditioning, or so I thought, until I turned it on to find out that it too, like me was sick and moody. At some moments, it felt great, pumping out clean and cooling air, while other times it just went to sleep, snoring away, letting out the occasional blow of lukewarm air like a cat coughing up a fur ball.

None the less we had air conditioning so I was grateful for that, and besides our view was nuts, small islands right in front of our deck, clear blue water as far as the eye could see that was moving all while I stayed put on solid ground, even in my state I did all that I could to grasp for something I was grateful for. Once we got settled in I jumped in a cold shower and planned to just lay down and chill on the bed while Josh went out to explore the island and grab a bite to eat. On his way back Josh brought me some veggies to eat but it was so hot with the manic A/C situation that I kept taking showers in an attempt to cool down. I wish at the time I could have had a positive outlook on my situation but I must admit, it was lame. I desperately wanted to go in the water, to take the bike ride that we had signed up for, but I simply couldn't move, I was exhausted and felt like a slug who had salt poured all over him in the hot sun. I did my best to embrace how I was feeling instead of trying to push it away and only prolong what my body was going through.

A few hours later I woke up from a nap feeling a little better so we jumped in a kayak and floated around the bay. Being the trooper that I am and not wanting to pass up a chance to film some cooking videos on the island, we started scouting out various little nooks that we paddled up to. The hope was to take out some of our veggies and spices, a few utensils, the camera and tripod and film something intimate and special. But by the time we got back from the ride I was so drained that we decided to do it on the deck of the bungalow. Unfortunate I know, but I was still proud that I stuck to the plan of filming, not letting the heat and how I felt change what we had set out to do. Sometimes you have to stick to things and push through no matter how much your body is telling you to abort mission. It felt good to be sitting outside but my energy was so drained, I didn't have my usual spark to jump around and be animated on camera.

Seeing how I wasn't myself and comparing that to how I know I could be on camera, I felt ashamed and not good enough, I knew it was mostly from feeling sick and struggling in the heat but it still got to me. Hearing these thoughts of self-doubt was one thing, I gave it airtime, let it play out and do its worst, but then, after a few minutes, I made the executive decision to push through and stop feeling sorry for myself.

Josh set up the tripod so it was looking out towards me with the sea in the background and as we started to film a group of younger, likely college aged, girls who were staying next door to us came outside and asked, "Do you have a blog or something?" We said no, but told them what we were working on, and how though our plans had changed because I wasn't feeling well, we were trying to make the best of it. At first, they thought that I had simply partied too hard the night before and was extremely hungover, but I assured them that was not the case. I had been so stuck in my world of battling sickness and heat that I even forgot the very notion of drinking. Josh and I aren't really drinkers anymore, aside from the occasional cocktail or glass of wine on a romantic date, but for plenty of people coming to an Island means busting out those shots and beers, I get it, I used to have the same urge but it has long since passed ever since I became aware of the damage it was doing to my body. Don't get me wrong, we appreciate a fine spirit here and there, but never for the sake of getting drunk. The sheer notion of a hangover alone make's excessive drinking an afterthought.

Sarah, one of the girls in the group, upon hearing what we were doing, was really surprised and interested, "That is so cool," she said, "my brother has a bad peanut allergy and has always been too terrified to travel to Asia, but with a book like this he would be able to travel."

Wow. I was completely taken abake. To attempt to create something needed in the world out of our own hopes and dreams is one thing, but to actually hear of someone who would benefit from it while we were in the process of creating this project and sharing our story felt so nice to hear, it felt like even though I was having issues with the heat and hormones, even though I was feeling beat down and maybe a little hopeless, that the universe must have heard me and was reminding me why we were on this journey in the first place, creating this content to give others hope to live their dreams, to explore the world, to do something they have always wanted to and overcome their fears of why they couldn't. I'm not pretending that my journey will be exactly, or anything like yours, but if there is anything that I can offer you it's the possibility that you can do anything, even if you've been taught throughout your life that you can not. With some planning, some creativity and a drive for something great, you'd be surprised what you can create in the world.

After our side conversation we sat on the deck, Josh wielding the camera, me making fresh summer rolls with the rice paper we had bought in Hanoi, and a mixture of ingredients we had cooked the day before. They turned out to be some of the best I have ever had, I wrapped those little rounds of heaven with some cooked cabbage, fresh thinly peeled veggies and roasted peanuts for crunch, plus I whipped up a little chili garlic sauce that I made in a coconut. Needless to say, they were delicious and satisfying.

Once we finished up I showered and we headed to dinner. Along the way, as the sun set, the island looked majestic. I was clean, the temperature was cooling, and I was starting to feel alive again. We stopped by the ping pong table and played a quick game, I was laughing my head off, I felt like a kid, it was such a blast.

When we arrived at the dining area I saw that it was a family style BBQ dinner buffet with a wide array of dishes. When we got there everyone was in line to get food and though my first thought was wondering what I would be able to eat as it turned out I had a special safe plate of food that the chef made for me. It was things like this that truly made me feel special and cared for, like things were continually flowing and working out in unpredictable ways. Yes, in moments I was definitely a drama Queen and a bit of a big baby with the heat, hormones and blah, blah, blah, sure, that was all true, but I knew I was also a trooper and did all that I could to rise above, and that I was getting rewarded for that with this lovely night with my boo.

As we sat at a bamboo table decorated with flowers and candles, full moon floating above our heads, the romantic ambiance was off the charts, which for Vietnam was not the norm, as it's not typically in the culture to show affection. Needless to say, Josh and I were taking full advantage of this, we were both bubbling with joy, holding hands under the dinner table, exchanging glances and giggling like little kids. We were on an exotic island being served a magical meal in a majestic place, regardless of what else had happened to me on the trip, we were so blessed and knew it. As we blessed our food in front of our other diners, two sisters; Katy, the chef from San Francisco who recently relocated to Kentucky, and her sister Fern, we struck up a conversation. We spent hours talking about food, cooking, and what having a strong community of support means to us and chatted about how special and important gatherings are around food with loved ones. It was really nice to have a commonality that was rooted so deeply in passion and pure love. That doesn't happen all the time so when it does it's pretty nifty.

With full bellies, and the feel good feelies, we left dinner for a moonlight stroll along the ocean. Honestly it was the first night where we both felt good and it showed, there was that spark, the same spark that we had before I got sick, before we found out that removing my IUD and having what I now know to be called the mirena crash, would throw all my hormones out of whack and make me sick for weeks, if not months. Like the Incredible Hulk coming to a little kid's baseball game and hitting the ball out of the park, into the sky and beyond, our connection that night was ever expanding into the infinite.

The next morning, we packed our things, got back onto the small boat which took us onto our previous boat and we sailed home. During the journey home, we were told that there would be a cooking class on board and that we would be making, sort of ironically, spring rolls. Being professional chefs, or cooks, or whatever you want to call us, Josh and I were all too familiar with making spring rolls, heck we had been making them most of the trip, but we understood that it was a class for everyone and that for most people it would be a fun and new experience.

As it turns out the word spring roll has a variety of meanings depending on the culture. In Vietnam, they typically use rice paper when making any sort of roll. Typically, summer rolls are the fresh rolls with lightly soaked rice paper and fresh yummy fillings inside. Spring rolls can mean a few different things. At some restaurants, a spring roll may refer to the fresh rice paper roll, just like a summer roll, or it may refer to a fried roll that uses a wheat dough instead of rice. In the case of Vietnamese food, it typically means a combination of the two, they wrap the filling in rice paper and then fry it up.

In the cooking class, which consisted of the teacher going through the steps while about 30 people huddled around him, and then letting each person have a go at rolling the filling he made in the rice paper and frying it up, I hoped to get a chance to try out the spring roll. Unfortunately, this was not the fresh vegetable kind of spring roll that I had hoped it was, instead it was made of a filling of vermicelli noodles, some cooked vegetables, salt, pepper, and an egg, with an option to have ground cooked pork as well. I asked them if I could have one without egg seeing as how I was allergic and for some reason they said no. I was rather confused as to why it was such a big deal to leave out the egg, but as I later found out the person cooking felt that the egg was necessary to bind the ingredients together when frying, which I understood.

It brought up an interesting point for me. Often when someone is taught the "proper" way that food is supposed to be cooked, the very idea of changing things up to them might be unthinkable. Josh and I are in the business of always changing things up, always trying new things, always pushing forward, but it's not like that for everyone, depending on the culture you come from, if tradition stands above all else, the very nature of change is a tough pill to swallow. Sure, it was frustrating at first and I felt a little left out, but at the end of the day it's nothing against me, he was probably just unaware that there was even another way to make the spring rolls without eggs. Sometimes when someone is unsure about your needs it's best to leave it be, for as much as it can be frustrating, if I had to choose, I'd rather have someone tell me they don't feel comfortable cooking for me over someone who disregards the severity of my allergies and just acts like they know what they are doing. Besides, we were visiting another culture, and above all else, we wanted to fully respect the

180

Vietnamese traditions and ways of doing things as best as we could.

Tip for Feeling Included

The more you spend time in a foreign country, the more you learn about the culture and can develop a feel for how you might be treated in each situation. Don't expect everyone to be completely open to helping you out, it's better to be grateful for the few that go the extra mile, than to get frustrated at the others who either don't seem to care, or, upon seeing your allergy card, simply wave you off.

Food allergies, depending on the country, may be a very misunderstood topic. For some people the very idea of changing up their recipe, even the very idea that you can't eat a certain food, might be unthinkable to them. We met plenty of people who were more than helpful and especially in tourist areas, willing to help, but if you are trying to really get down and dirty and go places where few foreigners have gone, don't expect everyone to cater to your needs.

Best to always prepare some food or be prepared to cook in these situations. Being aware, and knowing that there is a chance there won't be food for you is a great way to not get your hopes up and be let down. We had plenty of unexpected situations on the trip where I could eat something safe that was incredibly delicious, but I always made sure to be prepared with yummy food so I had something to munch on. That way, whenever someone went above and beyond to help, it really felt special.

After our spring roll lesson, we had fun with some of the crew. They were being silly and playing games with Josh, telling him to get on his knees and try to push a deck of cards over with his nose, putting a spoon in their mouths and whacking each other on the head, all before Josh had a pretend sparing session, like Bruce Lee, with one of the crew members, while all the

181

other people on surrounding boats laughed, pointed fingers and took pictures. They were a fun bunch and it really was a great way to cap off such an interesting adventure at sea.

When we got back to our hotel in Hanoi we found out that the train tickets to Da Nang were unfortunately fully booked but we found plane tickets instead that were very cheap so we booked a flight, packed up our things and decided to have one final night in Hanoi before leaving the following afternoon for the middle of the country. Little did I know that something would happen that night that would go against everything we had learned about eating safely on the street.

Chapter 15:

Street Food Sickness

That night, as I was starting to feel a bit better, being back on solid land and all, we decided to check out our bucket list of things to stuff our faces with that were special to the region. Josh had his list of special street food he wanted to try and me vegan and gluten free spots and treats. It was a great opportunity to shoot some b-roll for the gluten free travel videos we were still trying to make, even with all the changes, a way of getting extra beauty shots of local food, scenery and to really capture the night life vibe of Hanoi.

It was another hot one and sometimes when I'm hot I'm not all that hungry for solid food. I was craving veggie juice and so was Josh so we headed into the city to find some pressed fruit goodness. We spotted a quaint little juice cart on the side of the street that had a long line of people, always a good sign. All we had to do was point to the fruits and veggies we wanted and in a few minutes, we had an incredible energy booster comprised of colorfully loaded liquid nutrients. After drinking down our treat, I felt like I was ready for anything!

Next on the list was a vegan restaurant we had heard about online that had great reviews but by the time we got there it was already closed. There were several vegan restaurants in Vietnam, some we heard about online, others we stumbled upon, but even though vegan restaurants tend to be more consciously aware overall, you still must be careful as some places use a lot of wheat. The two biggest things to look out for in Vietnam when eating at a vegan restaurant are soy sauce and seitan. Soy sauce (which of course has wheat in it) is often used as a replacement for fish sauce in many Vietnamese receipts and seitan is a great substitute for meat (if you are not allergic to wheat). Seitan is made from vital wheat gluten, basically it's a celiac's kryptonite, and has a very meaty texture. You may be able to find soy based meat substitutes but make sure you are careful. Needless to say, that night we were out of luck on the gluten free restaurant front so I grabbed a second juice and sucked down another dose of liquid love into my body before wandering back off. I mean how can you pass up fresh juice when it's so hot and so cheap?

After my second juice, we stumbled upon an interesting looking bbq spot outside on a street corner that was packed full of locals and some tourists. All the tables had a heating device in the middle so you could continue to cook your food or keep it warm while you ate. Josh really wanted to try it so we sat down on these cute little kid red plastic seats, you know, the kind that felt like with one wrong move you might flip out your chair like a cartoon character.

Wanting to feel a part of the eating experience I took out some steamed corn that we had bought earlier for me on the street and like a gluten free gangster I asked for salt so that we could eat together. The way the restaurant worked was that there was a table filled with a never-ending selection of skewered things; marinated beef, chicken, shrimp, octopus, squid, mushrooms wrapped in beef, vegetables, tofu, you name it, they had it, all you had to do was select what you want, they would grill it up and bring it to you at your table with some dipping sauce.

Josh picked out what he wanted from the menu and we took our seats while the flames ferociously licked his masterful selection. It only took a few minutes for the food to arrive, the server turned on our mini table grill, putting the food on it to keep everything warm and while Josh ate his meal I chomped down on my corn enjoying the experience.

In the past I would have felt totally embarrassed to take food out to eat at a restaurant but now, even though I did feel a little unsure and a little self-conscious, my feeling for wanting to get over that was greater. I made sure not to listened to the little voice inside telling me to submit and told myself it was time to be a rebel and break all the rules! Besides, no one who ever changed history asked for permission (maybe they asked for forgiveness later on) and that's exactly what I was bent on doing. The best part, once I started eating, no one there even batted an eye at my corn, it really helped to remind me that I shouldn't overthink these kinds of things too much.

Tip for Bringing Food to a Restaurant

In the states, you will find that most restaurants are not so keen on you bringing food into their establishment. You might be able to get away with some small things, like busting out your own little chili sauce, but more than likely they will frown upon any outside food. This, however, I found was not the case in Vietnam. So long as Josh ordered a meal, no one seemed to care if I ate my own food.

I always did my best to ask, or at least gesture to the fact that I had outside food to make sure it was okay to eat, though I usually do now and ask for forgiveness later. But as far as I see it, if a restaurant can't serve me then what's the big deal if I bring something in on my own? Health standards and food laws are going to be stricter in certain places so it always helps to ask someone that works at the restaurant first if it is

185

okay, but you should never be ashamed of having to eat food that you know is safe instead of the food they are serving.

The next morning, something was wrong with Josh… He calls himself the iron stomach because he claims he can eat just about everything, and for the most part he has proven this true. However the Australian guy we met at Halong Bay with the stomach bug claimed to be the same way, that was of course until something happened. He wasn't sure what it was, likely the grilled squid he had the night before, but Josh couldn't seem to keep anything down.

The place he had eaten at checked out on our list of eating safe on the street. It had the busy line of people, the service was fast, everything was clean, but sometimes something can happen to you, even if you don't have allergies like me.

He said his stomach didn't hurt at all and he felt fine, but that literally the second he started to eat something, even drinking a little water, his body was like the exorcist purging everything out, only from the other side… The poor guy was slipping his brains out almost instantly the moment he tasted anything. I felt bad for him, I know how excited he was about eating the street food, and we did our best to make sure anything he ate was safe and clean, but even following all of our rules for the place we ate last night, something still happened. Sometimes things are going to happen while traveling and you have to be prepared.

It reminds me of a story, Heston Blumenthal, one of the world's most renowned chefs, Josh's food hero, was serving oysters to all of his guests at his restaurant The Fat Duck, voted one of the best restaurants in the world, one night for his immersive and mind blowing tasting menu. Somehow, and much to Heston's horror, everyone got sick, terribly sick with food poisoning. As it

186

turns out the batch of oysters that he got, though they were from an extremely credible and fresh source that he always bought from, were contaminated. It was a terrible blow to the restaurant which was considered one of the best in the world but luckily, he bounced back and is still considered one of the most esteemed and innovative chefs in the world today. Just goes to show, you can never really know what is going to happen, best to be smart, follow your intuition and know that if something does happen, so long as you are healthy, with some basic treatments, your body will heal itself.

That day Josh had planned to hang out with a fan and go explore some more food even though I told him to consider resting as I knew his tummy wasn't feeling good, and I wanted some time to myself to get a massage and do some self-care. When you are traveling with someone, whether a friend, family, or loved one, it's important to take some time to connect to yourself, have a chance to recharge and to refresh, especially if you are someone who, like me, is very giving of yourself.

We had had a massage in Ho Chi Minh but it wasn't all that much of a massage so I decided to splurge and really get a full treatment. Splurging in Vietnam on a massage after all isn't much more than $10, so I didn't feel too bad about it.

I found a place that had great ratings on TripAdvisor and opted for the full Thai massage. Holy lord, I was not prepared for what was about to happen... Imagine watching one of the fight scene's in Kill Bill, only it was happening on my back. The woman in charge of massaging me, though tiny in stature, was a beast of a masseuse, she was literally standing on me and digging into the fiber of my muscles with her feet. It was probably the most intense massage I had ever had, but it was also absolutely incredible.

After the massage, I found my way back to the hotel, not before getting lost in the myriad of streets because I saw a Bob Marley shirt that I knew Josh would want. When Josh saw me I could tell he was worried because I got back later than planned. He's so cute when he's concerned, but I understand because we were flying out that day and we didn't have much time, let alone a way to contact one another when we were apart.

Josh said he had a nice time on his little street food tour, walking around, checking out some street food and learning more about Hanoi, but that he wasn't able to eat anything, or keep it down for that matter. I was worried but Josh said even though he wanted to eat as much as he could, he took his stomach bug as a sign to take a break from eating. He admitted that on the trip he pushed it a little too hard, trying to eat everything that his eyes found intriguing, which was a lot more than he was used to eating. He felt that his body was giving him signs to chill out on the eating so it could have some time to reset and heal. Besides, he reminded me, we were heading to Hoi An, a serene city in the middle of the country, known for having some of the best food in Vietnam and he wasn't about to stop eating for too long.

Tips for Eating with Awareness

For as much as traveling with food allergies might feel like a burden, in a lot of ways, if you are smart, in some cases you might just be more safe than those who can eat whatever they want. Having food allergies helps you have a better sense of awareness for what you put into your body. Developing this awareness, though it takes some practice, is an absolute blessing once you see how important it is.

What started out as a very real need to make sure I was only putting in foods that my body could tolerate, has turned into something far more important and powerful for me. Learning how to be a conscious consumer, not just because you have food allergies, but because knowing what you put into your body is important no matter who you are, will change your life. Developing that sense of awareness, knowing how any given food might make you feel has so many positive health benefits.

It doesn't happen over night, but we have found that if you start cultivating a sense of awareness in the things you put into your body, becoming aware of not just what you are putting in, but how it is making you feel, you will start to see major changes happening. Sure, sometimes I feel left out that I can't eat everything I see, but once I remind myself that most of the food out there isn't even real food and that the food I eat is incredibly delicious and special, I don't feel so left out anymore.

Chapter 16:

We Got Mooned

The flight to Da Nang was simple enough. Da Nang, a far more untapped city than Hanoi, a place where you could get a sense of real local city life, without all the tourism, was in the center of Vietnam. We had planned to head to Hoi An, a beautiful and charming city near the beach, which was about 45 minutes outside of Da Nang, and then finish our last few days back in Da Nang before flying to Ho Chi Minh and then home.

As we drove towards Hoi An from DaNang, the sights of sprawling city slowly morphed into open air palm trees and a majestic view of a cool calm and blue ocean. Fresh coconuts and rolling around in the sand here I come! Did I mention I developed a new obsession with drinking fresh coconuts and then eating their flesh out with a spoon? Probably, but if not, let me just say, I probably had a fresh coconut every other day. Anytime I was feeling run down the healing tonic inside that hard shell always seemed to give me a nice boost.

When we finally pulled up to the homestay we had booked on online I knew our last week in Vietnam would be quite different. Unlike the hotels we stayed in, or the rustic homestay in the jungle, we had decided to stay in a place called My Moon Homestay. The pictures on Agoda, the site we used to book it, looked really nice, it had great reviews, and on top of that, Hoi An is not only known for their food, they are also known for having some of the best, and most affordable tailors in Vietnam. And lucky us, our host happened to be one.

The homestay was a beautiful place, big wooden open doors leading to a front room filled with rolls of fabric and mannequins wearing suits and dresses. There was a nice pool to the left, a luxury we had yet to explore in Vietnam, with the sun beating down as it was during the day, it's cooling waters were calling our names... By the looks of it the homestay looked newly renovated, the kitchen was open and simple, there was a nice outdoor seating area, in total it was three stories high, it was a huge. Upon arriving we were welcomed by Moon, the host of the homestay, a deliciously sweet Vietnamese lady who spoke in a broken english and tried her best to fulfill all our needs. We would later form a strong bond with her, but at the moment all we felt was a sense of being at home. Upon meeting her she told us that if we wanted to have anything tailored or made she would give us a very good price.

There were several reasons we wanted to go to Hoi An, one being that they are famous for their tailor skills. Just about everywhere you look in town there are tailor shops with a wide array of clothing and shoes in them, and at each shop the tailors can make just about anything you'd like. You simply show them a design from a picture or an actual article of clothing, they measure you, and then boom they are off to work, making adjustments along the way. Moon, in her broken English said it would be easiest to get work done with her, she was an expert tailor and since we were staying in her home we could easily get adjustments made.

As we were settling into our room we noticed there was no bathroom, it was down the hall. We asked Moon if we could switch rooms to one that had a bathroom build in, as we tended to use the bathroom a lot, and by we, I mean I, and she was more than happy to place us in a room one floor up that had its own private bathroom. What can I say, I like my toilet throne, especially in the morning, sometimes all you have to do is ask politely.

Once we got settled, the first thing we wanted to do was check out a restaurant we had heard about, supposedly the best restaurant in all of Vietnam for Vegan food. They were supposed to have a lot of gluten free options as well so I was excited! For the chance to share a meal that we both could enjoy at the same time felt like a big win considering everything going on.

We had found some vegan restaurants in Vietnam during our search, especially since there are a lot of Buddhists who often eat vegan or vegetarian meals a couple of days a month for holidays, but this place seemed to stand out the most amongst the rest as the reviews, claiming it was perfect for anyone vegan visiting the area. I was ready to stuff my face even if I was still feeling crummy, I may have felt like a bloating blimp, but I did my best to keep a positive outlook

We borrowed bikes from our homestay and pedaled through town towards our destination. Along the ride, we could get a nice feel for the town, it was a mix of residential roads and homes, local markets, large green fields and rice patties, all surrounding a cute town with loads of shops and restaurants. It felt somewhat like a lively beach town but it had an elegant sense of romance tickled along the streets.

When we found the restaurant we were searching for, we sat down and immediately started scanning through the menu. It was a really cool and eclectic menu, the vibe was more American than Vietnamese, it was cutely decorated, kind of like a par-hippie Californian cafe. There was a rather large variety of cuisines, ranging from vegan Vietnamese dishes to fresh salads, soups and anything else you could have wanted on a hot day. Typically, when in a country such as Vietnam, you want to be extra careful of ordering anything fresh and not cooked, especially things like salads that don't have an outer skin you can peel, upon reading reviews however, we decided to take our chances as everyone had only positive things to say about the salads and the rest of the menu.

We began to ask the waitress for some suggestions based on gluten free options that they offered and, much to our dismay, noticed that she was confused as to what we were talking about. Here we were, at a restaurant that promotes cooking classes, eating fresh, mindful and freshly organic food, and the waitress had no clue about gluten or what it even was. All the excitement and good vibes we came in with were instantly sucked out of the window. Every time I asked her about a dish she would say "yes, yes, I think that is fine, I think so." Now, it is from my experience from eating out that anytime a waiter say's "I think so," when it comes to asking what is in a dish, a huge red flag should go off in your head.

If you have severe allergies like me, the server and staff should always have a knowledgeable understanding of the food, ingredients, and overall sense of how the food is prepared, and if they do not they should easily be able to find out from the kitchen. You can't expect everyone to know about your food allergies, but if you can't find someone in the restaurant who does, especially the person cooking the food, best to move on and find something you know that is safe.

Mind you we are in a foreign country where food allergies are not a thing, so we have to give them a little slack on their end, but even so I can't give any slack on my end. We ended up ordering two salads just to be extra safe, triple checking to make sure that they were prepared properly, even going into the kitchen to watch as they made the food. Even so, we caught her on a mistake when she brought out the dressing.

Rule of thumb is never just dive into the food, no matter how hungry you are, the wrong plate could have been delivered to you by accident—that has happened to me a million times. So, we asked again when we got the food and even though she insisted the salad was safe, as it turns out the dressing on the side had soy sauce in it, even after questioning multiple times. Always follow your gut in these cases and ask as many times as you need to in order to feel safe. Again, I can't blame the restaurant, it wasn't toted as a gluten free place after all, just vegan, but vegan restaurants typically have options for gluten free, but, at the end of the day, you can never assume anything.

Dining Out Tip

If you are ever in a situation where you really need to eat, where you are starving, there is nothing else around, the food you found seems safe, but you are not 100% sure, well my first golden nugget of wisdom is that it is not worth it. My second being that if you decide to eat it anyway, just be sure to double and triple check with the server and the chef. There are a number of safety factors that go into eating out and the hardest one to control is cross contamination, but don't hesitate to ask about it or to look in the kitchen or ask to watch them prepare the food. Small things like making sure they are using a plastic and not wooden cutting board can help give you some peace of mind. Having extra things written on your allergy cards, information about how to prepare the food, not just what you can and cannot eat, is also helpful.

It may seem bold, it may seem crazy, or honestly just a pain in the tushy, it may even get you thrown out of the restaurant should you encounter the wrong type fo chef, that's happened to me before, but you have to be diligent, you know the repercussions. Honestly more times than not, the people working there are usually happy to let you see everything, especially in a country where food is their pride and joy.

Even though the food was good enough and fresh, and a vegan's dream in Vietnam, overall the experience was a bit of a letdown. All the reviews got us so excited to eat at a place that we heard was a godsend for Vegans. A lot of the reviews said things like "finally a place I can eat good food, it was so good I ended up eating here every day of my trip when I found it."

But in the end, we had no one to blame but ourselves. After all I got excited, maybe a little too excited, and assumed that jutst because the place seemed food conscious and was vegan that they would be able to make me something with ease. Sometimes the more we build up an experience, the harder we judge that experience and ultimately set ourselves up for failure. I should have known all too well from living in New York City that the hype of a place rarely lives up to the expectations you set upon it. More often than not the place that blows me away is the random one we stumble upon that is kind enough to make me something safe.

In the end, reading those comments about how good the food was and then having the experience we did, lit an even bigger fire in my belly to create something special for people wanting to travel and eat safely with food restrictions and allergies. There is always a silver lining in situations and in the end, you have no one to blame but yourself. We can sit around blaming others for not being "consciously aware" of our own situation, but what good does that do? How can you blame someone for lacking in knowledge, especially in an area that is very new to most people? You will only end up being hurt and let down, the best thing you can do is help someone to understand and educate them as best as they are open to being educated. For all I know it was that dining experience that helped our waiter to understand the severity of food allergies, maybe from here on out she will have a better grip on it. I like to believe that all things work out as they should and that people, with a little nudging, are open to change.

The next day we woke up early, got a nice workout in, a little blend of long stretching and yoga, and ordered breakfast at the homestay, which was included each morning. They had a variety of options broken into Americanized breakfast classics and Vietnamese special dishes, but they didn't have anything for me, so I just asked if I could have some fresh fruit. Moon sent a worker out to the market which was two blocks from her house. She bought fresh mangos (which were the best mangos ever), bananas and watermelon, and made me a nice fruit salad for me. To my magical salad, I added raw gluten free oats, nuts and raisins, which blended nicely with my chocolate protein powder mix that my naturopath had me buy to help cleanse my liver and body along with the herbal pills she prescribed to help me heal after the whole IUD situation. Weight gain, depression and hormone wackiness aside, I think everything I was taking was starting to help, I was ready for a full day out in town.

After breakfast, we headed into town to get lost and explore, taking a nice long bike ride down a scenic route. It was a beautiful place, situated between a beach and a river, there were heaps of tailor shops, food stalls, carts, and massage parlors everywhere. This was the relaxing Vietnam that I was looking for. Coming from crazy overpopulated cities, which I love, but living in New York City made us long for something else a little slower paced and quant. Hoi An was the perfect balance of Vietnamese life, with a peaceful and serene twist to it, plus it had all the goods of the city and all of the chill vibes of a cool beach town. We spent the day exploring the streets, popping in to tailor shops to see what the prices were like (insanely cheap off course), grabbing fresh coconut juice and fruit along the way, and when we were done we headed to the local outdoor market to pick up some food. The market was close to Moon's house and we figured it was a perfect way to cook for the week to make sure I was prepared with extra food, it's also an epic way to get to know the local food culture even better. All local markets may look similar on the outside, but once you get in and start exploring, you'll see a world of differences.

As we were shopping around the tent covered food stalls we realized that no one else was around, no locals, no tourists, and hardly any people working at the market. So, when we finally did spot some Vietnamese woman working at the market they really came after us aggressively, each stall we went by they yelled at us to "buy, buy" from them. It was hilarious because anyone of them seriously could have been an auctioneer, but it was also intense! We had to be careful not to get ripped off as it seemed like when they saw us we were their next money bag waiting to be emptied into their hands. It's funny, when we first arrived in Vietnam, with so much culture shock, everything seemed so cheap, getting ripped off wasn't even a worry, spending two dollars instead of one on the best bowl of soup of your life was almost comical, but as we adjusted to the culture, and knew the prices, we were on the hunt.

We had already learned a little Vietnamese, enough to barter with, as our local friends told us when shop keepers saw us the prices were hiked up. Plus, growing up in Ecuador I always loved and enjoyed the art of haggling and creating a bond between myself and the seller, to show them I wasn't the typical tourist, that I wanted to learn and be a part of it. Also, since we had already been shopping at all the other markets, we knew the general prices of things, and we knew better than to just trust their first price.

As we did our first-round walkthrough, seeing who had the freshest stuff and the best prices, we couldn't seem to shake these three ladies who were circling us, yelling at me like they were sharks in the water, being super aggressive, a little too much for me. I was actually starting to get scared because I didn't know what they were about to do, I felt like they were going to whack me or something but instead of backing down I got more and more aggressive, standing my ground as I realized what was really going on. When one of the woman grabbed my arm, and tried to get me to buy from their stall I ripped their hands off to make sure to let them know they couldn't push me around.

Let me just say I grew up with aggressive behavior while buying things in the markets of Ecuador and I could handle it but this was a whole new level I had not experienced. I felt like I was going to lose it because boundaries were being crossed when they started to touch me, pulling me this way. Josh was filming the experience happening, they didn't bother him, he didn't really seem aware of what was going on, just making sure he captured the interaction.

What should be noted is that I love learning new languages, I am fluent in Spanish and Icelandic, decent at Italian, and at this point of the trip I had picked up a lot of conversational language and words so I understood a good bit of what the ladies at the market were yelling at me. As they did their little dance they were laughing like hyenas to one other, try to see who could get the most money out of me.

When the biggest lady of the bunch came up to me, trying to pull me over to her stall, in a loud and authoritative voice, puffing my chest out like a puffin to appear taller and look strong I said "no, no," and I put my hand out in front of her face. At first they didn't change their song and dance but instead started to get louder, so then I got louder and I suddenly felt a fire being lit throughout my entire body and soul. I could sense the Viking in me coming out big time! I looked at all three of them and with both hands in the air, projecting the loudest and firmest voice I could, I said "this is not what I asked for, I want these bean sprouts and your price is too high, be nice and I will buy more from you and come often."

I kept going on and on in English like they could understand everything that I was saying to them, at first they just stared at me like I was a ghost but slowly they started to get quieter. Turns out the sterner I was with them, telling them that I wasn't some idiot foreigner trying to buy one thing, that I wanted to do a big shop and come often since we planned on staying a while, turned things around a lot. I also told them in my loud ominous sort of what I thought God's voice would sound like if he was pissed, that they needed to smile and play nice, that if they were going to act crazy that I wouldn't buy a thing from them. I don't actually know if they understood any of what I was saying or if they thought I was a raving lunatic about to go A-wall, but they started to smile and giggle at each other like they just saw the best comedy show of their life, belly laughing and patting each other on the back like they just won a soccer game. My growing fear ear turned to hilarity in a manner of minutes.

I felt larger than life, like I had just tamed wild lions, it was unlike anything I had ever experienced before, my blood was on fire, what had just happened!? As I looked to see where Josh was, he was cracking up, filming the entire fiasco with big wide eyes and a look on his face that I had never seen. They became more friendly and helpful then I could have expected after that. I knew that the locals were not accustomed to a foreigner shopping in their fresh local markets, but I never expected that kind of behavior, I guess humans will never cease to surprise me, myself included. I am amazed just how much changed in them once I firmly stood my ground.

The market was a large, open air market, with all the fresh vegetables and fruit you could imagine, along with meat and fish, all dirt cheap. I got a shopping bag filled with fresh mint, an amount which would have cost me around $12 in the states. The whole bag was cleaned, picked through, and the most flawless picturesque mint I had ever seen, the former food stylist in me was screaming with joy. And the price? All for 20 cents total, it was incredible. The quality of the food in Vietnam and the prices were unbeatable.

Chapter 17:

Using Your Hand as a
Cutting Board

After our wild, yet ultimately entertaining time at the market, we took our groceries back to Moon's home and she said that we could use her kitchen to cook whenever we would like. We told her about why it was so important for us to cook, how I had food allergies and that we were working on a book and filming the experience, she really seemed to love it and even offered to help.

Moon had a really incredible staff that helped her run her three-story home which was also a BnB and tailor shop. In Vietnam, fresh food was absolutely one of the most important aspects of daily life. Each day one of the workers would go to the local market and shop for food for that day. The very idea of buying ingredients to keep around wasn't even a thing for them, I noticed this when I opened the fridge and saw nothing but a few bottles of some sort of liquid for drinking.

One of the woman who worked for Moon, an older woman, in her early eighties, small, frail looking but tough as an ox, we simply called "Grandma," because we couldn't pronounce her name. She was so precious, she stayed with Moon and handled a lot of the cooking. Moon told us that she met her many years ago, and found out that she had no family, and was too old for a lot of work but was too proud to ask for help. Moon offered her to stay and live at her house and in exchange she would help cook food for the family. It was such a sweet story, everything that Moon told us about her life and what she did just made us have more and more love for her, it felt like we had found an angel on this planet.

It had been a long morning, we were getting hungry so we decided to prep some vegetables for lunch in the kitchen, doing our best to stay out of the way of Grandma and her young helper Suan, a quiet and shy, yet powerful in presence, Vietnamese woman in her mid-twenties, who was also cooking food for the family. It was then that we noticed something really interesting. about the way that they prepped food and cooked.

Rarely ever using a cutting board, the woman in the house would cut most of their food in their hand, peeling green beans, slicing up vegetables, all with the masterful skills of a pro chef. They would prep one thing at a time, never doing too many things at once like Josh and I were prone to doing. They would prep one vegetables, cutting and peeling it as necessary, and then cook it in a simple manner before placing it into a bowl on the table and covering it with a   mesh cover. Once they were done they would go on to the next thing. It was really inspiring to watch as they cooked with such focus and attention to every single ingredient they touched.

What we did find funny was as they cooked away, anytime we tried to do something that seemed perfectly normal to us, they would watch us in action, having fun as we cut our veggies up for a few moments, laugh with confusion, and then walk over to us, pleasantly shove us out of the way, and start doing it for us, as though we had no idea what we were doing and that they would do it right for us.

It quickly became obvious that they were less interested in learning our way and more interested in showing us their way, as

202

though it was the only right way to peel the green beans or anything else. It was an incredible and humbling experience, the way they would hold a cleaver in their hand and cut the veggies in the other hand. Just hand, knife and ingredients with such agility and precision that I had never seen outside of a professional French kitchen, where even they were using cutting boards.

The more we watched the more we understood what their food culture was really like. Each morning someone would go out to the market, buy only what they needed for that meal, maybe that day at most, come back, prep each ingredient, cleaning, cutting, one by one, and then one by one they would cook each thing, slowly, carefully, precisely. It was really special to watch, we learned a lot about the Vietnamese culture by staying at their homestay, something that was missing when we stayed in hotels cooking for ourselves.

With the help of the staff we made a simple but delicious meal. We were using inspiration from some things we had seen and ate the day before. One of the most noted was the fresh mint that they eat in Vietnam. Typically, in the states if you eat mint you would pull off the leaves, maybe give them a chop and throw some in something, but in Vietnam their mint is so good and so fresh that they eat it like whole leaves of lettuce, but even more so they leave it on the stem and you eat whole little bunches of mint. We made a salad with shaved carrots, a ton of fresh mint, and a simple chili-lime dressing, it was refreshing and delicious. When you are cooking such fresh food, you really don't need much at all, the ingredients really sing for themselves, and when put together in the right way create a symphony in your mouth.

After lunch, we took a walk to town and managed to find a soothing massage place that offered couples massages. We had been in Vietnam over two weeks and had hardly gotten to take advantage of the super cheapo massage prices, I mean we are talking under $20 for an hour and a half massage. When we booked our massage they first gave us a mini foot bath. Our feet soaked in a bath of warm water with lemongrass, cilantro and other fresh herbs. It was divine. The massage itself was very relaxing, not nearly as intense as the Thai massage I had had before, but it was nice to relax with Josh in our little oasis.

That night we decided to do a little more exploring to find the heart of the town. We were already in love with Hoi An but we knew we hadn't seen the main spot in the town yet where we were told was one of the most romantic places in Vietnam. After walking for about twenty minutes we started to come up to the canal that ran through the heart of the city.

When we found the area we had heard so much about we were amazed. It was a picturesque charming and quite romantic little town, it reminded me of other charming cities like Paris and Venice but with a Vietnamese twist. There were a ton of restaurants along a serene river with small wooden boats that you could hire someone to row you around in for a cheap price. Everywhere we looked we saw endless food vendors but most magically we saw the beautifully colorful and vibrant lanterns being sold on almost every street corner, something they are famous for in Hoi An. It was like being transported to another time.

As we walked to the middle of the town square, calming wind blowing in our face, lanterns lighting up the sky, we randomly ran into some people we had met at our homestay in the Mekong Delta, a friendly Australian family with 4 little kids who were rambunctious and adorable. They told us about a food tour that they did where an Australian man who had been living there for years takes a group around and has them taste over 100 things, they also told us about a great vegan restaurant that they ate at (luckily not the place we had gone to the day before), and how we would absolutely love it as all the food was traditional Hoi An food served vegan style.

Excited to stay on our journey and to find a romantic place, we said our goodbyes and kept walking around the town, crossing the water by way of a cute bridge. Hoi An was starting to feel like the gem of Vietnam, it was peaceful and romantic, something we had yet to see on our trip. Honestly in other parts of Vietnam even holding hands with your partner felt like a little too much PDA, but in Hoi An, the charm and the romance was in the air so we didn't care about showing affection to towards one another, I felt great and I wanted to show my love to my partner.

I wasn't hungry but Josh wanted to eat some dinner, I think he is always hungry, so we found a spot that looked interesting called Mango Mango and sat down to grab a bite. They had an extensive menu, the restaurant felt a bit more high end, fine dining than we had experienced on our trip, almost like a NYC restaurant with some sort of fusion menu. Josh ordered some small plates of goodies.

When the food arrived he seemed to really enjoy it as I took in the sights from our outdoor table overlooking the water. It was the first time in a while where I felt like I could just sit back and people watch as I sipped on my tropical passion fruit drink.

After dinner, we walked around some more, stopping at little stores to buy cheap and cute little trinkets as gifts for friends and family back home. They had the most incredibly affordable and awesome stuff to buy, you know, things that you have no real business buying but can't help it because of the price.

Too many amazement Josh really stepped it up. Here I thought I was the haggling Queen but when we found a stall selling what they claimed to be real pearls, something I had wanted since Halong Bay, I saw a new side of my partner.

The man told us the price was $15 which I didn't think was all that bad considering he showed us that the pearls were real but Josh shook his head and said no, too much, I want for $5. The man said "no, no, way too much, this is real pearl," and Josh said, "no I want it for $5." The man kept going lower, 12, 10, 8, but Josh said no. I started to whisper to him that $8 for pearls was really good, but he said no we can get it lower. Finally, as Josh stood his ground the man shook his head and said that it was too low and he could not do it. I was starting to get bummed because I wanted the pearls but Josh wouldn't let up, perhaps taking a note from my market haggling, and whispered to me that we should walk away.

To my dismay we started to walk away and said no thank you. Then, halfway down the street, Josh said "wait for it," and to my amazement, within moments the man was running us down saying "okay I do it for $5." I was speechless, we bought two pearl necklaces, one for me, and one for my friend who I would be seeing in San Diego after.

Tip for Haggling with Vendors

No matter what you think you are going to do, when you start shopping around in Vietnam and start seeing just how cheap the prices are, you are likely going to buy more than you set out to. While my first tip is to do your best to limit yourself, really think about what it is that you want and what you truly need, my second tip is that most street vendors who are willing to give you a bargain will let you know it very quickly.

If you go to purchase something and the vendor says "I will give you a good price," or "How much do you want for it?" that is always a great sign that you can really haggle the price down. Don't feel bad or convince yourself that it's already cheap anyway, the truth is, anyone willing to haggle is already overcharging their prices way more than you can imagine, no matter what they tell you. They aren't going to sell you something and lose money, if they are willing to go low from their original price, chances are that original price was market up super high in the hopes of getting an uniformed tourist to just buy it.

The moment they are willing to bargain throw out a number that is much less than the ask. Maybe they want the equivalent of $15 or $20 for a necklace, okay great, offer them $3-5. They will likely wave their hand, shake their head, and say that it's way too low, tell you how $20 is already a very low price or that it's real pearl and so on and so forth. That's okay, at this point you can offer $5 and say that's as high as you can go. If they say that it's too low the best thing to do is say no sorry and start to walk away.

At this point you have options. What may happen is the person selling will say something like "okay fine, you give me $5," and then you get the price you want. I can't tell you how many times we started to walk away from a deal only to have a street dealer run after us trying to make our original deal work. The other option, if the person doesn't come after you, is to make one final counter offer, maybe you offer $8 and see if they take it. Remember, you can always go back and pay the original price if they are not willing to budge, it doesn't hurt to try and walk away and see what happens, but regardless it's rare that you find a place on the street that sells something unique. Typically for every one craft or jewelry souvenir shop you'll find 100 others selling the same stuff, some might even have much better prices than the first one you found.

After trying our hand in some haggling we headed back to the homestay to get some rest so we could have a nice day of exploring the next day. When we got back we told Moon that we loved staying in her place so much that if they had room we would like to extend our trip and spend the whole week in Hoi An. She was happy to hear this and said that they had space for us every day except for one night, a night we would end up staying at another homestay reminding us just how warm and hospitable it was staying with Moon.

Moon, little did we know, had only been in the homestay business for 2 months, it was all very new to her, she had been a tailor for 25 years with a huge crew, doing quite well for herself, and decided to rent out her huge home to travelers. We had no idea, she was such a natural, so sweet and accommodating, the type of woman that you know was born to be a mother and angel to all those she encountered. She was endlessly fascinating to talk to, even if she was still working on her English, I learned so many things about Vietnam and life in general whenever we struck up a conversation.

Yes, finally, Hoi An was really starting to feel like the gem of Vietnam, our happy place. The food was fresh, the people were nice, the romance was serene, things were looking up, it looked like the end of the trip was going to really come together and make up for some of the rougher days I had. Everything was going well, that was, until I woke up the next morning and felt sicker than I had the entire trip.

Chapter 18:
Motorcycle Madness

To much dismay, the next day I woke up feeling really sick, I didn't know what it was, but I just felt terrible. We had planned to go scuba diving which I had been dying for Josh to experience, that weightless, timeless magic of being underwater... Most definitely one of my favorite sports for such a long time, ever since I got over my life long fear of sharks, but I just couldn't do it, I felt too crummy. Being sick is one thing, but being sick under water and dealing with pressure changes—no, I had to cancel our plans, it was too dangerous.

As the day went on things went from bad to worse so we made the decision to stay in Hoi An for the remainder of the trip. Often when visiting a country, especially one that takes over a full day to get to, it is easy to want to try and go everywhere, see everything, and do everything that you can possibly imagine. We had considered going to Thailand and Laos, something a lot of folks do when visiting S.E Asia, but we decided to stay in Vietnam and be fully present with all the beauty that Vietnam had to offer. There is so much diversity just within Vietnam, within each city even, so much to see, so much to learn, it made sense to stay. We had also been traveling so much throughout the trip we realized that staying in Hoi An was a welcome retreat to just be, to relax, to process such an adventure filled trip.

★Tip for Traveling★

Often when you travel there is this pull to want to go and see everything. You are already so far out, across the world, why not see as many countries and places as you can right? I'm not saying you shouldn't but more often than not I hear stories about friends who come as a tourist to a foreign country with a strict agenda, often times part of a tour guide and while you may end up with some great photos and detailed information, are you really getting a chance to be present in one place?

For some people traveling with a tour group is comforting, and for that matter it is great, but if you really want to get a feel for what everyday life is like, to really get to know a culture beyond its historical landmarks, to know what present day life is like, well then, find a place that you want to go and try to limit how much travel you do. Going from place to place every 2-3 days can also really be exhausting. But hey, to each their own.

I took the morning to stay in and rest. As much as I would have liked to go out I was finding that sometimes taking it easy in the morning would give me enough energy to go out later in the day. It was hard to stay in and relax, being somewhere I had always dreamed of being, reading a book didn't quite seem fulfilling, but I kept reminding myself it was for the bigger picture of the trip.

As the day progressed and my plan to rest worked, seeing as how I was starting to feel better, I thought it was a great chance to eat some delicious food without pushing myself too hard so we decided to try out that Vegan restaurant we heard about the night before.

When we arrived at the restaurant there was no one else around, likely because it was an off hour. It was a cute little place with maybe 10 tables or so and books lining the shelves. After a few moments, a man walked out and showed us to one of the tables before handing us a menu. Right when I sat down I politely asked him to look at my allergy card to which he had no issue understanding. What a relief. I can't tell you how much pressure melts away anytime I can tell that the waiter understands my allergies. The man felt extremely confident and even started pointing to things on the menu that were safe for me to eat.

We ordered a passion fruit "mocktail" along with a banana blossom salad, a spicy grilled tofu dish in a banana leaf, and much to my surprise, they even had a vegan and gluten free version of a famous dish you can only find in Hoi An, White Rose. If you have a chance to try White Rose you absolutely must, it is comprised of a gently steamed rice flour dough, almost like a super light and delicate dumpling with a filling which is typically made from shrimp, meat or, in my case, veggies, topped with crispy shallots and a fish sauce, chili, sugar and garlic dipping sauce.

This chewy cloud of heaven literally disappears from existence in your mouth leaving you feeling like a million bucks. The version we had was all veggies and the dipping sauce, sans fish sauce, even left me feeling really satisfied. The banana blossom salad was also extremely delicious. It had a bunch of fresh herbs in it with peanuts and a tangy dressing. If you have a chance to try banana blossoms I suggest you do, they are really hard to find in the states and such a treat for us anytime we saw them already cut up into thin strips at the market. The tofu wrapped in a banana leaf really minded me of eating a scrumptious curried steamed fish, the whole tofu was stuffed with mushrooms and veggies, it came out pipping out and we couldn't get enough of it.

We spoke to our waiter, who we found out was the owner of the restaurant along with his wife who cooked all the food and we went off in delight, complementing their skills until we ran out of nice things to say. It was really magical, to get to sit down and eat a special meal, especially after having not the greatest experience at the first restaurant, really meant the world to us. Just goes to show for as much research that you can do online, trying to find great places to eat, sometimes you discover the true gems from word of mouth or simply stumbling upon them.

After our meal we headed home, I washed off, a shower always making me feel centered again, and then we decided to take a bike ride before seeing the sun go to sleep. On our bike ride, feeling the wind blowing gently on my face, I couldn't help but feel grateful to be out of my room, sucking in fresh air, admiring the majestic scenery every which way that I looked. Paddling through the rice paddies, calm and serene as it was, we spotted some wild water buffalo. Josh, being the adventurous guy that he is, started approaching them, getting closer and closer, which of course was making me a little nervous.

As my heart started pounding, unsure of what Josh did, or didn't know about these mammoth wild creatures, I convinced him to back off, saying that they could be aggressive and attack, after all, some wild animals can be quite unpredictable.

We jumped back on the road and slowly made our way to the beach, a small local beach that was lined with a few simple restaurants and an area where you could park your bike for a small fee, along the various street vendors selling unidentified delicious treats. We parked our bikes, grabbed two chairs on the beach, ordered an extremely refreshing coconut drink (with just enough booze in it to share) and sat back as the sun slowly melted down into the horizon.

We didn't drink that much on the trip but the moment felt right to celebrate a magical, even if at times nightmarish, adventure with my love. As the sun set and the afternoon sky turned into a palate of bright pink and purple glowing clouds before fading into nothingness, we sat back, sipping our drinks, holding hands, and simply smiling.

Josh, getting hungry, (I swear he is somehow always hungry) ordered some delicious looking grilled squid with a spicy dipping sauce to cap off the night just before we jumped on our bikes and headed back home. Forgetting how fast the night sucks the light out of the sky we were forced to bike back in the pitch dark. I will admit, it was a little scary, biking down that long open road, which only an hour ago, was illuminated and peaceful, as it now felt dark and a little bit creepy. Funny how your mind can race as soon as the light is gone.

Josh, sensing my nervousness, blasted Bob Marley on his iPhone to lighten the mood. We peddled our little butts of, singing "don't worry about a thing, every little thing is going to be alright," until my fears melted away. After a few minutes, I had a sudden burst of inspiration and so I signaled to Josh to pull over as I grabbed him gently, swinging around, dancing in the road, no one around for what felt like miles. I knew this moment would sew into my heart forever as we turned a small fear into a sporadic romantic trip as we danced with the stars over our head. I felt full of radiance and health once again, my sickness was gone, life was restored once again.

The next day Josh booked us a surprise trip to take a motorcycle tour around and outside of Hoi An in the countryside. What I didn't realize was that not only was it a private tour for just the two of us, it was an all-day event, and on top of that it was freaking hot outside. I tried to tell myself that I was up for the trip, riding on the back of a motorcycle, zipping

213

through the countryside, it all sounded awesome, but to be honest I wasn't feeling as great as I would have liked to.

Not wanting to let Josh down, I decided to keep my physical state to myself, hoping that by not saying anything my nausea from the morning would miraculously disappear. I figured that the fresh air would do me good, besides, what could possibly go wrong in nearly 100°F heat, on the back of a motorcycle, on the open road, hormones all out of whack?

When the bikers pulled up, we were a little caught off guard. Josh had found them on some random website online (he has a knack of doing anything he can to avoid the simple, safe, booked by your hotel tourist day trips), so when the two middle aged Vietnamese men pulled up in full leather getup, clearly not the cheery and talkative tour guide type, we couldn't help but look at one another with part confusion and part laughter.

We strapped on helmets (thank God), hopped on the back of their motorcycles, and sped off towards our first destination. The first stop we hit was My Son, a must-see place if you visit Hoi An. My Son, according to Wikipedia; is a cluster of abandoned and partially ruined Hindu temples constructed between the 4th and the 14th century AD by the kings of Champa. The temples are dedicated to the worship of the god Shiva, known under various local names, the most important of which is "Bhadresvara".

It was absolutely stunning; the ruins were unlike anything I had ever seen before. What I did not realize however was just how hot it out would be in the open air. Hoi An during that time of year was quite hot during the day but we hadn't realized it because of how much time we had spent inside due to me not feeling well. As we came to find out most locals, similar to what I remember growing up in Ecuador, would wake up early in the morning to work, sleep during the day when the heat was unbearable, and finish up work as the sun cooled down in the afternoon.

As we walked around, snapping pictures at each ruin that amazed us more than the one before, I did my best to chug water and pour it over my head to keep cool as I munched on some fresh fruit. It helped but the sun was scorching, even with our little umbrella, it was beating down on us like a giant stomping on an ant.

I swear the fresh fruit was my saving grace in Vietnam, it was so fragrant, so delicious, you could suck a fresh mango right through the skin without even peeling it, I felt like a vegan vampire biting into its victim, drinking all of its life force, as it gave me a few moments of renewed vigor and excitement to keep going.

Our drivers had allotted far more time than we needed, or could really handle in the sun, so when we got back after about an hour of exploring they were a bit confused but happy to take us forward.

We jumped back on the bikes, trusting that wherever they were taking us was where we wanted to go, and we were off. We drove for about thirty minutes before coming to some beautiful rice patties which at first I thought was wheat fields. It was in that moment that I realized I had never actually seen rice growing up close. The drivers pulled over, we got off their bikes and they took us into the rice fields. We approached a unique looking metal box that had a long open square tube at the top. One of the drivers walked over to a pile of picked rice and began smashing it inside the tube. As we found out this was how the locals separated the dried-out rice from their stalks. He gave us some to try, it was super fun whacking the heck out of the rice, hearing the small rice grains dropping into the bin below. Learning the process of how rice was harvested only made me appreciate the majestic grain even more.

After shucking, I think that's what they call it, the rice for a few minutes, we got back on the motorcycles and continued. We zipped through winding pathways around endless fields of vegetables, noticing the dynamic growing systems used in Vietnam. Their agricultural system was fascinating, they had these large wooden structures resembling little huts that act as little grow houses for zucchini and a myriad of other veggies. The veggies would dangle over the structure leaving the dirt floor barren enough space for a farmer to get underneath and harvest their vegetables.

We saw people picking fresh peanuts, which we got to try, and learned how locals would dry the peanuts, rice and chili peppers in the sun, right in the middle of the street. I'm not kidding, everywhere we drove we saw huge tarps of red chilies sun drying, right next to the vehicles driving by, sometimes a wheel would even ride right over the tarp!

After about another 30 minutes of driving we came upon a small river as the dirt road disappeared. The drivers got out, went over to a man working nearby and after a few minutes of speaking to him he drove us onto his small boat which took us to the other side of the river. It felt cooler on the river, I couldn't help but pull a titanic as I yelled "I'm the King of the world!" at the front of the boat.

When we got to the other side of the road we headed down the dirt path eventually winding up in a small town where we pulled into a local restaurant which we were told served a famous chicken and noodle dish that Josh had never heard of. As I declined the meat and started to inquire about the ingredients used in the dish our guides seemed really confused. It seemed as they couldn't understand, for the life of them, why I would not want to eat meat. As it turns out they had never had anyone on their tour deny the food before, this was their first time with someone who had food allergies and who would not eat meat, I was really starting to feel like an alien, and I was fine with that.

We spent some time sharing with them about celiac disease, talking to them about food allergies in general and how I lost my craving for meat in recent years. Lucky for me, because of the layout of the open kitchen, and for the fact that they only served one dish with a few variations, we were able to talk to the chef, using our translation card, and find something safe that I could eat. We could watch as they prepared the food, being sure that there was no cross contamination, noting how simple and fresh the food was.

I had a nice bowl of fresh rice noodles, fresh herbs galore, and chilies with white vinegar, it was the perfect meal—light, fragrant and delicious. It's amazing how satisfying something so simple can be with a little chili, some citrus or vinegar and fresh herbs. Josh seemed really stoked on his chicken dish as well so it was a win, win all around.

Following our meal our guides took us to an amazing and private waterfall on top of a mountain. There were no other tourists anywhere in sight, they even told us not to tell anyone about it, not even our hosts, it was that untapped, hence us not sharing the name here because hidden gems are meant to be found by the adventurous traveler.

At that point, leading up to the waterfall, I was about ready to go home. Being on the back of that motorcycle, exposed to the harsh sun, I was feeling really dehydrated and wasn't sure how much longer I could make it. Luckily at the very instance that I dipped my toes into the healing water at the entrance towards the main waterfall I immediately started to feel a bit better. Jumping in with all our clothes on, because we didn't bring swim suits, felt incredible, like any sick feelings were suddenly washed away.

Feeling the power of the waterfall, I felt the healing energy that it was giving us, as though it knew we were coming and had the perfect remedy for my ailment. The main waterfall was about a ten-minute hike up, it spilled into the smaller pools below, the higher we climbed, the more we heard its powerful roar.

When we got to the top of the waterfall there was a group of young Buddhist monks, ranging in age from about 12 to 18, all playing around and laughing with one another. They thought it was funny that we were there, clearly out of place, and kept pointing and laughing at us, getting a real kick out of our very presence. Without speaking a word of English one of the monks came towards us and challenged Josh to a swimming race. First one to swim to the base of the waterfall and back would be the winner. They were all laughing so hard, I wasn't sure if it was some kind of practical joke or prank, but before I could begin to think about what was going on Josh tossed his shirt off as he accepted the challenge.

The young monks, still giggling and pointing at one another, used hand signals and various gestures to try and explain the rules before counting down from three to start the race. When the race began Josh, very seriously, jumped in the water and began swimming ferociously as though it were the Olympics, determined to not be shown up by a teenage monk. The monk however was not much of a challenger, he was barely paddling, doing his best to even stay up in the water, as though he could hardly swim.

Josh smoked him out of the water in seconds, every one of the monks roared with joy at the spectacle and fun of it all, they were so sweet and innocent. When Josh got out of the water to dry off they spoke in very broken English and asked if we were married. We simply chuckled and said maybe one day before thanking them and heading on our way.

It was the perfect afternoon together, enjoying all the joys of nature, getting to see a very real piece of Vietnam, I was grateful to have the energy to do it, even if I did push myself a little too far. We had one more place to go, the Marble Mountains, but after speaking to Josh we decided it was best for me that we start heading back. When we told our drivers we were ready to head back they seemed a little confused. Josh was worried they would think that we weren't having fun but after he told them we would still pay in full, they seemed to ease up.

On our way back we made two quick stops. The first one was at a Vietnam war memorial. Now, I must say, some people from back home told me before the trip that they were worried about going to Vietnam because of the Vietnam War that had happened not all that long ago. We had briefly wondered this ourselves, but after doing research, and being in the country, we found that there was virtually no prejudice or issues with anyone towards Americans. As we came to find out, the Vietnam War was a small blip in the history of Vietnam being invaded by other countries, fighting war after war, and that in general Americans were welcomed with open arms. There may be some people of the older generation who had more strings attached, but we didn't meet anyone that seemed upset about the war or us being in their country, all in all the Vietnamese people are a very welcoming and open culture. .

When our driver pulled over to the memorial and got out he told us that he lost his father in the war. I could tell that it was very emotional for him, and while for a second I wondered if he had any negativity towards us being Americans, thinking us responsible, I soon realized it wasn't about that for him, he was simply proud of his dad. It was a touching moment as I too had family who fought in the Vietnam war. It was a great reminded that at the end of the day we are all people, often in war there is no intrinsic right or wrong side, people simple fight to protect their family, to protect their culture and country.

After taking a few pictures and learning a little bit about the war from his side, he took us to one final place to grab a refreshing drink of freshly pressed cane sugar juice that we gratefully gulped down before heading back to our home stay.

It was an emotional day on many levels, seeing the ancient temples in the immense heat, learning how rice was harvested, eating a fresh meal, cooling down and recharging in a beautiful waterfall, learning about the war, I was truly grateful that I had the strength to make it through the day, but when we got back it all came crashing down. I could hardly hold my head up, I felt my body shutting down, I needed to get in bed fast.

Chapter 19:

Sick in Paradise

The next dayI had hoped to have the momentum I'd had a couple days prior when we biked to the beach but when I woke up I could hardly hold my head up long enough to eat a meal. Everything took a huge dive, I felt extremely dizzy and heavy, my ears were clogged up like they had been days prior to us leaving for the trip, I felt like I had vertigo, I could barely stand, I felt like death.

Josh enlisted Moon to help us find a doctor, which she did in a matter of minutes and within an hour a doctor had arrived to check me out. He was a short and intense Vietnamese man who came with nothing but a bag with some of his medical gear.

When Josh asked him how much it would cost the man practically yelled at him saying "why you care about price? I check her out, or I don't, we don't talk about price, we talk about her". I think it freaked him out a little bit but he said he understood and let the man proceed.

We told the doctor my symptoms, he checked my blood pressure, listened to my heart rate, asked me a few questions and gave me some pills to take, for motion sickness and a few other things. I told him that my biggest fear was flying, we only had four more days left in Vietnam and the very idea of traveling 24 hours home feeling this way really freaked me out. I was starting to feel trapped, would I be stuck here forever? No, of course not, but that's one example of where the mind can go in distress. Besides we were supposed to fly to California where I was set to speak at a large gluten free expo, I couldn't bare missing that.

221

The doctor really wasn't sure what was wrong with me, he thought it might be heat exhaustion or sun stroke, but wasn't sure. On top of that most of the pills he gave me, even though I never like to take pills, had ingredients that I was allergic to so as nice of it was for him to pay a visit, it didn't do all that much for me.

One of the other guests staying at Moon's Homestay, Suzy, a sweet middle aged Australian woman traveling alone offered me some acetaminophen to help with my fever, splitting migraine and the rest of the pain in my body. As I came to find out, it was basically the same thing as aspirin which at this point I was willing to take to help take the edge off the intense pain that I felt. It helped a bit but at the end of the day, all I could do was rest up.

Over the next day or so I felt like my illness was going back and forth, at times I would sleep for ten hours, having vivid dreams where Josh told me that I had ruined the trip and that because I got sick he left me and went back to the states saying that I was burden and he didn't want to be around me. What a nice dream let me tell you, and one very telling of where my mind was at.

Waking up from a dream like this only made me feel more sick and freaked out, almost as though I had lost the one person I loved more than anything. What made things even worse was that when I would wake up, frozen in pain, hardly able to call out, and see that he was gone, I would only get even more freaked out and even started to think, in my delusional state, that he had actually left.

In reality he had only gone downstairs, or to the local market to get some fresh food and coconut water to help me feel better. When he walked in the door with a smile and fresh fruit, I would break down in tears at the sight of him and tell him what I had dreamt as he calmly would listen to me and sooth my fears with the reminder that I was loved and deserved to be taken care of and that that's what you do when you love someone.

For me this was a relatively new experience that I had never had in any other relationship and a revelation that someone could love me, just for me, even if I was sick, considering most of my early years I felt like a huge burden anytime that I was sick, always being made to feel that I ruined family trips.

When I would start to calm down it seemed like my illness would slowly start to clear up allowing me to shower and go to the bathroom by myself and even sit at the balcony in our room and look out at the greenery just below while chatting with Josh. It came in waves, things would clear after a nap and then start to get really intense. I felt hopeless, depressed. During this time, Moon was like a mother hen checking in on Josh and I frequently to see if we needed anything. She was so concerned with my wellbeing, I had never experienced such kindness and love from a stranger. While I felt terrible, feeling her support, and Josh's, really opened my heart and made me realize for the first time in my life that people loved me just for me, that they didn't care that I wasn't scuba diving or running around and doing wild things, but that they just loved me for who I was no matter what, both stranger and my partner alike. Sickness can be such a great teacher.

To help keep me fed, Moon would make me rice porridge to try to help keep me nourished. When I tried to tell her that I could not eat it, she reassured me that it had nothing in it that would make me sick, by now she knew everything that I could not eat as we had explained it to her while sharing meals. But I had a feeling that it was made on her non-stick pan that she

223

prepared wheat products on and when I asked she confirmed it indeed was so I was not able to eat it. When I tried to explain cross contamination, she didn't really understand. Not wanting her to feel bad for all the work she put in for it was such a kind gesture, after trying to explain I would simply say thank you and Josh would eat it.

Non-stick Pan Tips

While some people are more sensitive than others, I like to be extra careful and avoid eating from any non-stick pans that have had wheat cooked in them. Non-stick pans can develop small scratches in their non-stick coating if not used properly and wheat can hide in there believe it or not. We brought our own non-stick pan as well as bought a regular pan to cook in. A lot of places you will eat in Vietnam will not use non-stick pans as their main source of cooking pan but it's always helpful to find out or even just ask to see the kitchen if you want to be extra careful. Seeing that they are using plastic cutting boards is always a great sign as well as stainless steel or cast iron pans. Don't hesitate to ask the chef to clean out his pans regardless of what type they are just to be extra careful. When in doubt don't chance it, you can always eat some freshly peeled fruit or some rice steamed in a rice cooker.

The next day was mostly me staying in bed and doing my best not to lose my cool, it was hot, I felt like hell, and I was missing out on the end of a trip that I had always wanted to go on. That really was the hardest part of the trip for me, being in a place I had always wanted to go with what was seeming like more and more the man I wanted to spend the rest of my life with, this trip was really solidifying that in my heart, but being stuck mostly in bed. As a result of me not feeling well Josh would stay with me to keep me company, he would read me books, we would listen to music, hang out and go through pictures from the trip, and occasionally he would go on little outings only after my relentless pleads for him to go out and enjoy himself. I felt like we missed out on half of the trip because of me. No matter how I tried to spin it, it felt depressing, like I had weighed down the entire trip and ruined things for the both of us. It reminded me of growing up and being sick a lot as a child, always feeling like the burden of my household, costing my parents lots of money, worry and time. I hated feeling like a burden but I had no idea how to change it.

For as sick as I felt, what made things even more challenging was that for the brief moment that I was still feeling good I went a little nutzo custom designing and drawing out 18 articles of clothing with Moon. From shirts to shoes to dresses and even a sick suit for Josh. Because of this Moon was coming around and having me try on things to be adjusted, even if I didn't feel great I was determined to come home with a new custom wardrobe that I felt good about. While I was excited to be getting back in fashion mode, I always wanted to have my own clothing line and used to design custom aprons, having to work on the clothing did add a lot of unwanted stress on me which in turn delayed my healing process.

And to make matters double worse even though we had decided to stay the full week in Hoi An and ditch out on Danang, Moon did not have any rooms open for the next two night so we had to move to another homestay and then come back to her place for the last few days.

Chapter 20:

Lost My Mind at the Beach

Josh found us a nice place not far but it was no My Moon homestay and that night when we checked in there was NO HOT WATER. I had to take a freezing cold shower already feeling like crap, it did not add a nice touch to the already shitty day I was having, regardless I was trying hard not to turn into a big grumpy pants. On top of everything we had planned to do some filming at the beach the following day and I really just needed a win.

Sometimes I tended to forget that we were filming the whole experience due to my not feeling so great and not wanting to be in front of the camera, but I was hellbent on getting some footage at the beach since we had already missed out on some big opportunities, so we sallied forth.

We spent the first night getting to bed early so I could be rested up for our shoot, hoping and praying I would feel okay. The next morning Josh went out, bought some veggies and prepped as best as he could. I had no idea what we would be filming but he packed all the gear and food and we slowly pedaled our bikes to the beach. As I started to pedal something in me started to shift, I began to feel alive, in fact I felt so alive I almost felt like I was on drugs, it felt like I was tripping out or something, it was crazy, I had so much energy. I was all over the place like a little kid on a sugar high.

We got to the beach just before the sun was getting ready to go down and sweep out of existence for the night, purchasing one whole tiger crab for Josh on the way in that I told him I would even cook for him. When we walked onto the hot sand we saw clusters of local Vietnamese families having a good time, swimming, playing, lots of small fires rumbling away, groups of people grilling and selling all kinds of smoked meats and a variety of local dishes. Everywhere we looked vendors were set up casually on the beach, tending to their fires, selling food and drinks, it was magical, and for a change I was feeling fantastic as I took in the night.

Unsure of how this would all play out for us as we were one of few locals on the beach, we rented a large blanket to secure our space, took out our little gas burner and cooler filled with food, Josh set up the camera and just like that I was hosting my own little cooking show in the middle of a beach, surrounded by locals. That is where things started to get interesting.

Little did we realize that because of the gusts of wind on the beach our little burner was barely working, the food was sitting in the pan getting lukewarm at best. Thinking quick we put some of our things around the burner to shield it from the wind, some towels, our cutting board, we were desperate. A word of caution, be careful what you put close to your burner should you end up in a situation like ours as towels could easily catch fire. We were very careful, but still it crossed my mind how embarrassing it would have been trying to cook next to the locals on the beach and lighting our towel on fire Mrs's Doubtfire style.

When we finally got our burner going it felt like a huge accomplishment, after all, sometimes you really have to celebrate the small things, especially when you really need a win. As for the food I had no idea what to expect but I felt like I was on such a happy wave from conquering the burner that I felt even higher on life.

As our little carrot and squash skewers started to fry up in the pan and Josh hit record on the camera I started to get really silly; talking to the food, making jokes to the camera, shaking the salt like I was holding down percussion for a salsa band, and before I knew it a crowd of Vietnamese people were watching me and taking pictures of me. Funny thing, when you are a tourist the locals don't notice you, you are more likely to take pictures of what you see, but in our case, we were doing something so foreign to them that they started taking pictures of us and looking around at our little set up.

It was all fun and games until these two shady looking beach patrol or cop guys came up to us, watching intently, with very serious looks on their face, standing uncomfortably, a little too close to us, giving off confused and uncertain looks like we should not be doing what we are doing.

Instead of acting weird or scared of them I invited them to come over and to try the food, which in turn kind of shocked them. All of sudden they weren't feeling it and quickly walked away as we continued to eat and be goofy together. I finished cooking the veggies which we kept simple so we could dip them into some freshly made turmeric, ginger, garlic and chili sauce and then I did something that might just freak anyone vegan out a little bit.

On the way in to the beach we had seen these ladies selling fresh seafood, all very cheap, right by the beach. Thinking back on our trip, aside from some steamed clams we had with Kelly, we hadn't cooked any meat or seafood for Josh. Sure he had eaten a ton but I wanted to do something special for him. A big part of this journey wasn't just about me being able to make things that I could eat, but showing ways to share meals with your friends and loved ones to create connection.

I could see Josh eyeing these beautiful tiger looking crabs and though I wasn't sure how I would feel about cooking something alive, I knew how much Josh would appreciate it, he had been such a trooper and I wanted to show him my appreciation. I put the crab into our pot, covered it and ran him over to the ocean. When I got to the cool water I filled up the pan with some sea water, a trick I learned from my scuba days that really gets the essence of the sea into the crab, and then we boiled the crab with some turmeric paste and other spices until it was fully cooked through.

As the sun went down Moon and our friend from the hotel showed up to join in the feasting. We had invited them as it was one of our last days and we wanted to spend some time connecting as well as get to know them a little better. We sat around and ate the food which was again simple but oh so satisfying. Josh said how deliciously sea salty and tender the crabmeat was, how it was life changing and that I should consider trying a little bit.

Reluctantly I put a little crab flesh on my tongue thinking I would potentially be transported to heaven and maybe even be un-veganed as growing up it used to be my favorite food. As a child, I would visit my god father Bobby's house and he would take us crabbing and then afterwards prepare a feast with bowls of hot butter and lemon juice. As a little kid, it was ecstasy, but now, having been a vegan for so long it just felt wrong and yucky, I spit out the meat saying sorry to the crab for wasting his flesh but thanking him for the offering.

As day quickly turned to night Moon, who continued to surprise me, said she goes swimming at 5am every morning in the ocean. As she was saying this she started to take her clothes off, revealing a bathing suit underneath and jumped in the water, so naturally like she was a little kid, so we all jumped in not wanting to miss this grand opportunity. It was dark, it was magical and I knew it was a moment we would never forget. It was also a little bit creepy, swimming at night, my mind kept racing to Jaws and how sharks feed at night, but I pushed those ridiculous thoughts out and splashed away in the water, feeling grateful to be alive. Oh, what a day that was.

Chapter 21:

The Long Road Home

The next morning, much to our relief, we got to move back into Moon's place for the final few nights. My sickness was back and forth during this period, sometimes it was awful, being bed ridden due to vertigo and not knowing if I farted whether I would poop my pants, yes even my stomach started to hurt and I had only eaten safe things we prepared, while other times I could do just enough to take a short walk into town with Josh. We explored the beauty of the town, focused on eating freshly made stuff that we prepared at Moon's house, and I did my best to take it easy and relax.

We did manage to find a dish that is considered extremely special, Cao Lau, a noodle famous in Hoi An. Josh had tried the dish one day while I laid in bed and said it was fantastic but that it wasn't safe for me. To our surprise, one day at the market we noticed that they were selling the fresh Cao Lau noodles used in the dish and after finding out that they were safe, snagged some to take home. Often times at local markets you can find all of the ingredients you need to prepare nearly any dish, already prepped out and ready to go, from curry pastes, to fried garlic, spices, and fresh rice noodles.

What makes Cao Lau so special is that it's made in a small town near Hoi An that uses a secret recipe that requires water from a special well and ash from a local tree. You can only get this dish in Hoi An and nowhere else, so needless to say I was over the moon that we could buy the noodles and try our own version.

After eating I managed to work up just enough energy to help Moon finish my clothing designs, she made us a ton of amazing clothing and we got some shoes made as well from a friend of hers. The shoes had some issues and it was in that moment that I realized even in times of sickness I am not a pushover. The lady making the shoes came with my designs to Moon's house to show me what she had made. Some of them were great, but most of the shoes were not what we had discussed. I imagine this is the case sometimes and that when people design something they simply think that even if their design isn't what they wanted that it's cheap and they should just go with it. Oh no, not for me, I told her that this was not what we discussed and that she would have to make them the correct way otherwise I would not be buying. Being clear and honest is important to me, if you want something done correctly you have to stand for it.

The last two days went by slowly, we didn't do all that much but after I got used to the fact that I would not be doing all that much I tried to do my best to enjoy it. On the final day, I made sure to really just relax. I hated not being able to go out and explore Vietnam, being stuck in bed it was hard to stay put but I did the best I could as I knew I needed to feel okay to make the flight back.

On our final, however uneventful day, we said goodbye to Moon, I shed many tears, I knew I would miss her, she was like a mother to me in those days, taking care of me, being super sweet, we promised her we would return someday. We made sure to make enough food that we could take some on the plane as well. I always like to have my veggies on the plane as well as little snacks since you never know what sort of food you will have access to in the airport. We had a long journey home, first driving to Hoi An to Da Nang, then flying to Ho Chi Minh where we had an 8-hour layover. After that we had to fly to China, wait about 6 hours and finally take our 15-hour plane ride, not home but to San Diego.

Before the trip, I was looking forward to San Diego, we would spend our final week in California, starting with a few days in LA and then driving to San Diego to spend time with my bestie and soul sister Shelia who was running the Gluten Free Expo. I would get to do a cooking demo and speak in front of hundreds of people about my journey in Vietnam. Yes, before the trip I saw it all very clearly, I would be coming back, ready and eager to share my adventures with the crowd at the Gluten Free Expo, to inspire them all to overcome their fears and go travel overseas, it was going to be great.

But that was before I got sick, before I discovered that having my IUD removed would send my body into a downward spiral, that was before my trip turned out far different than I could have imagined. Now, all I wanted to do was skip California, fly home, plop in bed and sleep until this terrible feeling went away.

Tip for Traveling Home

When you are heading back home bringing food back can be a bit trickier. In our case, we had to fly from Da Nang to Ho Chi Minh, then to China and finally back to the states. The issue with the return flight is though you can bring food on your first flight, once you arrive in another country you may have to give it up as you pass through immigrations. I would always suggest that you ask if you can bring the food instead of assume and throw it away. It's always smart to declare any fresh or cooked food you are bringing through the border, they might take it but, it doesn't hurt to ask and mention that you need it because you have food allergies.

A lot of times when people at the airport hear "food allergies" they simply nod their head and let you through.

Another important thing is to have a translation card for any other country you are passing through. Luckily, we had a Chinese translation card, otherwise I could have been screwed. On our layover in China we found a Starbucks and I was getting excited to get a little drink for a caffeine boost and asked to add soy milk, knowing it was safe at Starbucks as it always had been. After I ordered I thought better and decided to ask them to check the box just in case and as it turns out the boxed soy milk, similar to the one back in the States in appearance, actually had barley in it. That was a close call. We managed to get some freshly steamed greens at the airport as by that time my food had been sitting out too long and the flight home actually had some great steamed veggie options for me. A little ground chili, some nice salt I brought and I was set for the ride home.

Chapter 22:

I Can't Do It

When we got to Los Angeles I was starting to feel a bit better. Maybe it was being back in the states where the weather was a bit cooler and less humid, or maybe it was something else, either way I was glad to be one step closer to home. The plan in California was to spend a few days with Josh's cousin, explore the area, and then drive down to San Diego for the expo.

We mostly took it easy in LA; family dinners, exploring K-town, cooking some nice meals, checking out the beach one day. I knew I wasn't 100% and wanted to rest as much as I could to conserve energy for our time in San Diego.

When we finally got to San Diego I was excited to see Shelia, it had been so long. I hadn't spoken to her on our Vietnam trip so I was dreading having to tell her what really happened. She was so excited to hear all about our travels and a bit surprised when she heard about how sick I was. We had a great time connecting but there was much to do before my big talk. In Vietnam, our original plan was to spend the last week going over my talk, relating it back to how awesome it was traveling in Vietnam even with my food allergies, how I ate well, felt great, you know, all the stuff I had planned before. Seeing as how I could barely move on my last days and when I could the last thing I wanted to do was sit around and do work, I came to the expo completely unprepared.

The morning of my big lecture I panicked. I couldn't do it, I was unprepared, I didn't feel well, I wanted to walk away. I told

Josh that morning that I wasn't doing it. I told him that he could go down and tell Shelia that it was off, that I just didn't have the energy to do it. I wasn't prepared and I felt like crap.

Josh did his best to give me a pep talk, told me that I was a natural on stage, that the preparation was the trip, but it didn't matter, I had already made up my mind. I told him it was off and that he could tell Shelia if he wanted to but that it wasn't happening regardless of what he, or anyone, said.

When he left, my eyes filled with tears, I sat in the hotel room alone, praying for a sign. My trip had been ruined, my big moment to shine and share with the world all that I had learned was destroyed before me, it had all been a waste. I was ready to pack my things and get out of there but I decided to pause one last time, go deep within and pray.

Suddenly, praying to my higher self as well as my father, praying that he would be there with me, something sparked inside and lit up my entire body with such clarity and fire that I can't even begin to explain. In that moment, I could see everything very clearly, that the universe was using me as it's vessel to give people a deeper faith and love within themselves and to remember that they always have a choice, that their life is a blessing, food allergies or not. I texted Josh that I was going to do it and rushed down to the stage where we had already prepared food the day before that I would be demoing and sharing with the audience.

The moment I started my talk I was channeling from a place I had long forgotten. Words were coming out of me, people's eyes wide open as I spoke of passion, deep love, overcoming adversity and sickness. How my life, all of the good and bad thing,s had led me to this very moment, how I was able to share my story in the hopes of inspiring others to live their life to the fullest and not use their food allergies as weakness or crutches but to find the true blessing in all that you are. You see, while food allergies can feel like a burden to most people, I am forever grateful for having food allergies. I have managed to use my allergies to my advantage, I am a great cook thanks to so few restaurants being able to cook for me, I eat better than I ever have, thanks to really expanding my knowledge about how great vegetables could be, I take care of myself, I have created incredible bonds, and I am so much more aware of the foods I put into my body now, making sure they not only taste good, but make me feel good. .

After the talk, I never had such a long line of people waiting to talk to me, everyone kept saying how I left them moved and inspired. People were coming up to me throughout the rest of the expo telling me how I had changed their perspective on how they were living and how they saw that they could change their lives. It was in that moment that I realized I had created a new perspective of empowerment and freedom for those who had come. Suddenly the trip all made sense, the sickness, the battling, my entire life even came into complete clarity. I was here to help others, those like me who had gone through similar things in their life, suffered both physical and mental trauma, I was here to help them shine, to see the good that comes in the most unexpected ways and how we can take failure and strife and turn it into empowerment and positivity.

Chapter 23:

2 Years Later

It's crazy how things unfolded after the Vietnam trip, so much changed, exploded and shifted within me, the heart expansion that followed was beyond unexpected, I guess you could call it a spiritual awakening, but regardless I am forever grateful.

When we got back to Brooklyn we worked hard on creating the campaign to raise funds for the whole trip, for the book and the filming which was very exciting at first but very draining, confusing and time consuming as we had no time to decompress. When we launched our indiegogo page, we didn't raise even a quarter of what we needed which was rough because we had taken a month off of work for the trip. Leaving my bank account empty and feeling like a failure because I didn't know how hard it would be to run the campaign or that I was also hormonally still out of whack since taking out the IUD before the trip left me in a downward spiral of depression and not at all inspired to finish the work.

When work kicked back up I was ridden with shame and guilt that I became stuck and unsure of how to finish the book. During that time I found myself slipping deeper and deeper into depression. Josh did his best to be supportive but he had just signed a TV deal to host his own show with his brother on MTV so he was getting too busy to work more on our project.

On top of that I went to the doctor and found out that I had adrenal fatigue amongst some other issues and rest was prescribed as well as medication. I threw out the prescriptions and started therapy since I didn't know what else to do about depression, and to top it off I started to grieve my father's loss all over again. Time passed and soon it was Christmas, the book was still not finished, and I felt like I was running out of time, constantly falling off the deadline I had set for myself and all the incredible people who had helped support the campaign.

Being that it was Christmas we had a break from work and Josh surprised me by booking us a trip to Austin, Texas, a place we had both been dying to visit. The day after Christmas he proposed on his knees over a candle lit dinner he had made for us, taking out two boxes, one of a ring he had been making by hand for three months and the other a stand in ring he bought because he wanted me to have something that I could wear incase the ring he made did not fit.

The wedding, which will likely be a book within itself, came and went, it was a magical time filled with a mix of incredible memories, and terribly painful emotions that really put our relationship to the test, something that I am finding happens often when two families come together and two lovers create their own new first family. But the real test came when we decided to go back to Asia for our honeymoon, first stopping in Bali for ten days and then heading to Thailand for the last week and a half.

This trip was not only the best three weeks we had spent together going on adventures, cooking, learning, exploring, spending late nights talking under the stars, it was so much more than that. It was life affirming, for all that we had been working on in our hearts, minds and bodies to be whole and one with the world. We had successfully taken a trip, using all the tools we garnered in this book, and had the time of our lives, I never got sick, I didn't feel left out, we ate the best food I've ever eaten, and cooked the best food we've ever cooked. It was in that moment that we were reminded just how important it was to get this book out, to those that need that extra push of confidence to get out there and see the world.

Whether you have food allergies, celiac disease, or like to travel consciously, I hope that our journey together moves you. I pray that you feel seen, heard and loved, and that you remember you are not alone in this big beautiful winding journey of life, and that with some self-love, compassion, trust and planning, you can lead the most powerful inspired life you can imagine.

You deserve to be happy, to be loved, to be supported, not to feel like a burden or to feel shut down and isolated by what you can and cannot eat. I'm not pretending for a moment that traveling the world with allergies is easy breezy, but if you empower yourself with the right tools, I can promise you you'll be grateful for taking a chance and creating something new in your life.

If you do take that chance, that leap of faith, and have that trust, you just might return home renewed, happy and healthy. Trust yourself, plan well, be smart, I did and I'm here to say it turned out way better than I could have hoped.

Sure it was a challenge, at times I felt shame, guilt, got sick and upset, got lost many times and felt hopeless in my own mission, but in the end I found myself and the love of my life and hey, you might just too.

Note: If this book left you feeling empowered, inspired or happy we encourage you to pass it on or send a copy to a friend who just might benefit from this story . You don't have to have food allergies or celiac disease to use this book, anyone who has lost their way, is looking for their tribe, feels alone at times, or is looking to be healthy and happy while traveling can use this book as a tool in their life. Together we can change the world, one story, one page at a time, it starts with us remembering that each one of us is worthy, is lovable and beyond deserving. Thank you with all of my heart, I am infinitely grateful from here to the farthest stars in the milky way galaxy and back, to all those who have supported this book and its crazy journey to get here. This has been a true labor of love.

With a full + happy heart,
Jaquy Yngvason
www.jaquy.com

Chapter 24:

From My Partner's Perspective

Hello everyone, Josh here. First off, thank you for taking the time to read our story. We wanted to share this experience and though it turned out far different than we had imagined, it was an amazing and life changing experience. This book is for anyone that needs that extra push to take the rewarding risk that a life fully lived has to offer.

As the partner of someone going through such an intense experience, I thought it would be nice to express to anyone in a similar situation what it was like from my side. Truth be told, seeing Jaquy going through what she shared in the previous pages was heart breaking at times. Here you are, with the person you love, on the trip of your dreams, and you end up having to take care of them for nearly half of the trip. I felt terrible watching her like that, struggling, trying to push through when I knew in my heart she was only doing it to make me happy, trying to pretend like she was okay in certain moments when she was definitely not, just to not let me down. On top of that I was going through some major life changes myself, deciding if I wanted to quit my once life's dream and leave the band I had been with for 10 years, a band I started with a friend in college. My dream to be a touring musician was slowly fading away as I lost touch with the group, all while in the smack middle of intense negotiations for my first major network television show.

But all that aside, I would have just as happily spent the whole trip inside with Jaquy if that is what she wanted, she is everything to me and any moment with her is perfect no matter where we are (even those seemingly not so fun times.)

But as I write this, two years later, thinking back on that trip, I am reminded and shown just how far we have come, how far Jaquy has come. Truth is, though I didn't speak about it much to many people, there was a large portion of my relationship, early on, when Jaquy would get very sick. Times when she couldn't get out of bed, paralyzed from the neck down, couldn't move for days, shooting pains all throughout her body. Long stretches when she would be on and off the toilet for hours at a time, gut wrenching stomach pains, splitting headaches that plagued her whole day, cancer scares from numerous doctors, the list went on and on all from a mix of a few accidental gluten poisonings, and emotional stress and trauma.

This is really hard to admit, but there was a very real time in our relationship when I had to come to terms with the fact that I had married someone who had some seriously deep seeded health issues and that we would have to work through them, and deal with them together, most likely for our entire life. I can't tell you how many message boards I read, how many people I spoke with, who said that this was never going to change. And the scariest part is that I almost believed them.

Yep, I came to that very real possibility many years ago, that I fell in love with someone who would always be sick, even worried that it would only get worse and worse. But in the back of my mind I always knew that sickness was not really the life that we chose together. And while others projected their fears on me and their personal experiences, that they were not real, that what we had could overcome any sickness, all we had to do was trust one another and show each other that we were there for the long haul.

It was in that moment that a huge shift happened. Not only did things start to slowly get better for Jaquy's health after the trip, once her hormones balanced out, but we were able to work through a lot of deep seeded pain that we both struggled with and create a safe space to transform the hurt and fears in our lives together. We were able to create a new way of being for ourselves, one that had us showing up in a way that we could create anything we wanted for our lives, not live in our past hurt and fears.

Since then life has been incredibly exciting. Jaquy is a freaking health warrior who is not only healthier than ever, but one of the healthiest people I know. It has been truly incredible to watch her go from being sick on a weekly basis to never getting sick and being stronger than ever.

When it comes to food, the meals we make at home continually amaze us with how delicious yet simple they are. When we want to switch it up we have no problem finding safe restaurants and dining out, whether it be near our home, or when we travel around the world using the tools that we have acquired over the years.

As I make the final edits on the book, the amount of self healing through food, meditation, and a healthy lifestyle that Jaquy has gone through blows me away. And getting to do it together makes it all the better. But it's also the reason she is such a powerful transformation coach and positive life advocate, because she has been there, she dug through the trenches, went through hell to find heaven on Earth, she didn't learn about living a powerful life in a classroom, she lived it and solved the key to unlocking never ending abundant health.

We are beyond grateful to have the opportunity to share our journey with you. We want nothing more than to inspire you to get out there and live your life, regardless of what sort of fears or issues trouble you and hold you back. Take a moment think about what you really want for yourself, write it down, write down your fears and reasons for not following through, and then chuck those fears out the window and go live the life of your dreams. If we can do it, you absolutely can.

About Josh and Jaquy

Jaquy Yngvason, half Icelandic, half Ecuadorean, is an intuitive transformation coach and holistic food healer. She is on a mission to spread her passion for personal healing through her groundbreaking and transformative work.

Jaquy spent the better part of her childhood in sickness and pain, practically living out of hospitals, being misdiagnosed with depression, bi-polar, and brain tumors, only to find out years later that she had Celiac Disease and a number of other food allergies that were really causing her health issues. Driven to figure out how to heal herself, feeling as though the medical community had failed her, Jaquy started studying all things food and working with alternative modalities for healing such as Shamans, Medical Intuitives, Healers and more.

After graduating from Le Cordon Bleu and working as the head chef at a restaurant in Seattle for a few years, Jaquy grew tired of living off of epipens and Benadryl and learned that by working at the Food Network in New York as a food stylist and culinary producer, she could make food look amazing without having to actually eat it. In just a short few years she went from being an intern to a full on culinary producer and has gone on to work with top talent such as Bobby Flay, Aarón Sanchez, Paula Dean, Geoffrey Zakarian and Roger Mooking.

When her dad was diagnosed with stage three malignant melanoma, she started to implement her knowledge of holistic nutrition, personal experience and the Gerson Program to help him heal through whole foods, juicing, mediation and energy healing. After doctors saw the transformation that occurred during his treatment and were confused as to why he had such good spirits for his stage of cancer, Jaquy realized the powers of food. Unfortunately her father was too far along in his illness but before his passing he told her that her life purpose was in healing others through food.

Feeling that her true message was yet to be shared, Jaquy left her high paying and comfortable job and started focusing her energy and efforts on helping others like her, those that struggled with food allergies and eating disorders, to take control of their lives and develop healthy eating habits. She got certified in NFCA's Gluten Free Kitchen Program, completed Cornell University's Plant-Based Nutrition Program and went to IIN (Integrative Institute for Nutrition) to become an optimal living coach and even went on Food Network's 'Chopped' to promote Celiac disease and food allergies. From there she started speaking nationwide at allergy-free expos on living an abundant allergy-free plant based life.

Now Jaquy travels around the world working with others to help them find fulfillment in their lives through health. She leads workshops and retreats, speaks at public events and hosts a weekly woman's circle. She recently released a kid's book that she co-authored called "Super Dudes Eat Super Food" to help parents inspire their kids to love vegetables.

Using a plant-based diet, eating whole foods, and taking a mind, body, and spirit approach, Jaquy has cured herself from disease and illness that stemmed from misdiagnosed food allergies and has thankfully found freedom from depression, illness and her battle with eating disorders. She truly understands health and healing at the core, and it is her life's mission to help others to create and sustain a culture and environment of health, balance and thriving energy.

Josh Greenfield has been a professional sound and movement practitioner as well as a teacher of the creative art of cooking for over 10 years. What started out as a passionate hobby turned career as a guitarist and backup singer for a band called Canon Logic, later morphed into something quite different as Josh discovered the true healing powers of music and food. Growing up Josh was a terrible singer, he could not sing on pitch, hated his voice and when he spoke it was from a place of anxiety, often mumbling his sentences. He developed a technique to help anyone overcome their fears and past conditioned habits that hold them back from what their voice truly has to offer.

Josh also has a strong passion for teaching people how to cook and after being raised with a mother who did not like to cook and mostly served boxed, frozen, and fast food options, Josh started to cook for himself and learned the art of making homemade meals, using food as a vehicle for self exploration and creating community. Josh had spent years being sick to his stomach and suffering from terrible indigestion problems due to the quality of food he was eating.

When he moved to Brooklyn with his band in 2007 after college, immediately he started going through some major shifts in his life. Being broke and getting laid off from his job after the 2008 recession, Josh started cooking for himself and friends as a way to save money. Slowly others started hiring him to cook healthy weekly meals for them as well as throw dinner parties and before he knew it he was cooking for thousands of people around the city.

When his brother moved in to help out, a friend of theirs started filming their life and within a year they got picked up to be one of the first funded cooking channels on Youtube. After doing three seasons on a channel called Hungry, Josh and his brother decided to create their own channel called Brothers Green Eats.

Their channel now has over 1,000,000 subscribers and is designed to help people who struggle with cooking and are on a tight budget find the inspiration to get in the kitchen and change their life. He also co-created a TV show he hosted with his Brother on MTV that aired in over 150 countries and shot 31 episodes traveling around the world, cooking for major artists such as Ed Sheeran, Enrique Iglesias, Blink 182, Michelle Phan and D.N.C.E.

Since then he has been focused on helping people live powerfully through food and music and he teaches a movement and voice technique as well as curates music experiences to help people get out of their head and into their body while tapping into their inner ability to sing and speak with power, control and confidence.

Jaquy and Josh recently moved from Brooklyn to Denver to life out their life's dream and share their practice of conscious consumption both in person and online to help those in need find fulfillment in all areas of their life. If you would like to work with either of them or learn more about what they do please check out www.Jaquy.com for Jaquy's coaching practice, and www.YELMusic.com for Josh's music practice.